Sel

Born in Russia in 1954, Meir Schneider emigrated to Israel with his parents at the age of four. He underwent five eye operations without success, and at seven was declared legally blind. Years later, by means of eye exercises and movement therapy, he was able to read without glasses, and began work with other physically disabled people, receiving national attention for his work in the healing arts. In 1975 Meir emigrated to the United States to continue his studies and in 1977 founded the Center for Conscious Vision in San Francisco, then establishing the Center for Self-Healing in 1980. Schneider's work is now well known throughout the holistic health movement, and his unique approach to health care – the empowerment of the individual – is a message of inspiration and hope as well as a practical guide to specific exercises for everyone.

'In a most candid and heart-warming way, Dr Meir Schneider tells us about his experiences in dealing with his own severe handicap and those of countless others. As in homeopathy, acupuncture, and other forms of holistic healing, his work is based upon the application of appropriate stimuli to the natural healing powers of the body. He teaches us how we can improve our health, even recover from the ravages of degenerative and so-called incurable diseases. A book worth reading, full of thoughts worth taking to heart' – Leo Bakker, MD

'Meir Schneider's story has implications for all who go on a healing journey. His bodywork approach is the best I've experienced. Meir's courage and imagination in developing a new therapy have been an inspiration for my own work for a decade' – Ray Gottlieb, OD, PhD

SELF-HEALING
My life and vision

Meir Schneider

ARKANA

ARKANA

Published by the Penguin Group
27 Wrights Lane, London W8 5TZ, England
Viking Penguin Inc., 40 West 23rd Street, New York, New York 10010, USA
Penguin Books Australia Ltd, Ringwood, Victoria, Australia
Penguin Books Canada Ltd, 2801 John Street, Markham, Ontario, Canada L3R 1B4
Penguin Books (NZ) Ltd, 182–190 Wairau Road, Auckland 10, New Zealand

Penguin Books Ltd, Registered Offices: Harmondsworth, Middlesex, England

First published by Methuen Inc. 1987
Published by Arkana 1989
3 5 7 9 10 8 6 4 2

Library of Congress Cataloging in Publication Data

Schneider, Meir.
Self healing.
Includes index
1. Mind and body.   2. Exercise therapy.
3. Schneider, Meir——Health.   4. Blind——United States
——Biography.   I. Title.
BF161.S38 1987   615.8'2   86–20433

ISBN 014.01.9127.5

Printed and bound in Great Britain by
Cox & Wyman Ltd, Reading

Contents

v

Acknowledgments

This book took nine years to write. At times it seemed impossible to express in one volume all the aspects of the self-healing process: my own experiences learning to see, the underlying theory and philosophy of self-healing, and the stories of some of the people this work has benefited. I would never have undertaken this project without the direction and support of my spiritual mentor, Herbert Fitch.

When I began writing, I had just moved to the United States from Israel. My vision was still poor and reading and writing English was difficult for me. I decided it would be easier to dictate the book on to tapes and have someone else transcribe them, but even that was difficult because what I needed to say was so personal and deeply felt that it was frightening to share it with the world. My greatest help came from Hannerl Ebenhoech, a wonderful Austrian lady who acted as midwife to the book. For several months we held "writing" sessions, where Hannerl would come and sit with me, listening to everything as I recorded it. She said little, but her expressions and gestures conveyed love, understanding, and enthusiasm. With her support, it became easier for my story to flow. Even when Hannerl could no longer sit with me, I continued to feel her encouragement. When the tapes were completed, Hannerl transcribed them all, struggling to understand my limited English.

ACKNOWLEDGMENTS

After the book was typed we took a trip together to edit it, all 800 pages, but we both liked the entire manuscript so much that we weren't able to change it. However, the response from other friends, patients, and students, was totally unfavorable.

I thought about giving up, when Maureen Larkin, my close friend, who is also my patient and one of my better students, took it upon herself to rescue the project. Maureen, along with Margery Anneberg, an artist and long-time patient, spent two years putting my thoughts into comprehensible English and logical sequence. It was my unwillingness to allow them to cut much of the material that made their task all the more difficult.

In the summer of 1984, Nancy Wilson Ross visited San Francisco and through a friend agreed to read this manuscript. Her encouragement, along with her insistence that the book be shortened, made me realize that I had to write it again more briefly. As a result, we gave cartons of material – tapes. manuscripts, and literature on self-healing – to Deke Castleman, the managing editor of a nearby small press, who trimmed the book to a manageable size by removing repetitions and shortening the stories down to their essence.

The final rewriting was done in two week-long marathons by myself, Maureen, Margery, and a Zen priest named Arnold Kotler, who had worked in publishing and whose incisive questioning helped our editorial process immensely. During hundreds of hours, the four of us managed to recreate the spirit of the original tapes while polishing the form and further clarifying the content. At last we felt the book was ready, and to our great joy, the publisher Routledge & Kegan Paul felt the same.

I would like to offer my deepest thanks to these friends who made this book possible, and to many others too numerous to list. Special thanks are due to Muriel Wanderer, who patiently proofread several versions, offering valuable suggestions, and especially to Eileen Campbell, my editor at Routledge & Kegan Paul, who believed in this book.

Introduction

One evening last summer, I ran seven miles along the beach in San Francisco, from the Cliff House to Daly City and back. The air was quite cool, but the sand was warm from the day's sun. I felt carried along effortlessly by my feet, with no strain at all on any part of my body, my heartbeat just above normal and my breathing smooth and even. My eyes were thoroughly enjoying the glorious view of the ocean, the evening sky, and the hills of the city. When I reached the end of the beach, I sat down. Where my feet could no longer carry me, my eyes did. I watched the swelling waves, foaming onto the shore. I could see a gentle, sparkling spray covering the rock formations, which appeared like castles, caverns, and bridges. I inhaled the moist air and relaxed deeply, thinking about my family, about Israel, and especially about what it had taken for me to have this intense visual experience. From the very first, it had been to the sea that I went to work on my eyes, using the sun, the fresh air, the waves, and my own body as healing instruments. Tomorrow I would be returning to Israel for the first time since I had left nine years before.

My entire family met me at the airport. They had always discouraged me from practicing the "useless" eye and body exercises that eventually enabled me to cure my blindness, and they discouraged me from teaching the self-healing methods I'd discovered to others, even though it was leading to remarkable cures even before I finished high school. Yet, it was a joy to see them all, my parents, my aunts and uncles, and especially my Grandmother, the one loving soul who had encouraged me in this endeavor from the start.

I went to see Miriam, my first teacher, the woman who guided my first steps in self-healing. After searching for her home for a long time, I knocked on her door, and her voice came through, saying, "Who's there?" "It's Meir," I replied. "Who sent you?" she asked. I was stunned; she didn't remember me. "It's me, Meir," I repeated. "Well, who sent you?" At last she opened the door, but she still did not recognize me. "Miriam, it's Meir, remember? The one who cured his eyes from blindness." When at last she understood, Miriam had to clutch the doorway to keep from falling over; then she grabbed my shirt and began to shake me and hug me, laughing hysterically. She pulled me into the house and introduced me to her guests, still laughing. "This is Meir, the one I told you about. I can't believe it!" I found out then that some of those people had been hearing stories about me for years.

I lectured to several hundred people at the Vegetarian Society, the first organization to support and promote my work. Even the Secretary of Israel's Parliament came to the workshop which followed. One partially blind woman, who had never before been able to read print, was able to read some letters by the end of the third day, and several people with severe spine problems experienced relief after only one day. My old friend and colleague, Vered, was there, with Channi, a former patient of ours. They were both polio patients. Channi, who had needed a cane to walk when I first met her, told me that the cane had stood unused in a closet for the last ten years. They started to do exercises they had not done in years, and Vered's creativity blossomed, as it always had. She took my instructions as a starting point, and from there created a dozen new exercises of her own, finding the power within herself to move her weak leg in ways even she could not believe.

I showed people the difference between movement and exercise. Movement is the essence of life, and every movement brings new life to the body. The innate intelligence of the body is revealed through subtle movement – it is a tool to create every desired improvement. I encouraged people to discover and create exercises suited to their own bodies, as Vered had done. I was amused to see how different my Israeli students were from students in America. The Israelis were very boisterous, and everyone was an expert, explaining to everyone else what I had meant by what I said, and then yelling at each other for not letting me talk. I was the only quiet one in the group, and they all complimented me on my courteousness, something I am never accused of in America.

On the last day of the workshop we were joined by Miriam, my Grandmother, and my Aunt Nechama, who was trying my work for the first time. Aunt Nechama was astonished that after doing eye exercises she could read without her glasses, and Grandmother's pride was boundless. She had always supported me, and she was now able to see the fruit of her careful tending. Grandmother had suffered from heart trouble and swollen joints for several years, and was hardly able to walk when I arrived, not able to climb stairs without help. By the time I left Israel, she was walking by herself without difficulty, and she told me, "Meir, the best thing you could possibly have done for me was to heal yourself, because now everything you brought to yourself you are giving to me."

I have written this book in the hope that many, many others will also benefit from these simple discoveries: that the body needs movement and attention, that no ailment is incurable, and that hope should never be abandoned.

Part I

Growing up blind

Chapter 1

Savta

It was Savta, my mother's mother, who first realized that I was blind. This was in Levov, outside of Kiev, in Russia, soon after I was born. She observed me closely for several days, and when she was sure, she prayed to God for the strength and wisdom to accept this new tragedy – another handicapped descendant.

Both my parents are deaf. My mother, Ida, lost her hearing at the age of three, following an undiagnosed illness. My father, Avraham, was dropped by his family's maid when he was one year old, and he suffered brain damage which left him deaf. They met at a school dance in Levov, fell in love and married. My father's mother was so afraid they might have handicapped children that she slept in their room to prevent them from consummating the union. But as consummating a union is impossible to prevent, Mother became pregnant with my sister, Bella.

Bella was completely healthy. Thus made confident, my parents had another child five years later. I was born cross-eyed, with glaucoma (excess pressure in the eyes), astigmatism (irregular curve of the cornea), nystagmus (involuntary eye movement), and cataracts (opacity of the lens). In short, I was blind. My father was very busy launching his photography studio, and my mother, being deaf, felt incapable of handling the special needs of a blind baby boy

3

and an active five-year-old daughter. So her parents moved to Levov to look after Bella and me.

Grandfather had been arrested in 1943 by the Communist government, eleven years before I was born, for capitalist business practices in running a department store. He was sentenced to eight years in Siberia, and the government confiscated his large home, and moved seven families into it. After only six months in Siberia, Grandfather was released when all the Polish-born Russians in the camp were conscripted to serve in the Polish Resistance. But when the Polish general in charge learned that Grandfather was a Jew, he kicked him out. Although freed by this curious circumstance, six months of abuse and hard labor had broken his spirit, and he returned to his family a bitter man.

It was left to Grandmother to take care of me. My earliest memories are exclusively of her. When I was six months old, she took me on a train ride to Odessa, on the Black Sea, nearly 1,000 miles away, to see a leading ophthalmologist. The doctor examined me and declared that I would need surgery as soon as the lenses of my eyes were hard enough. Savta* tells me that I loved the train and that I hated the doctor. The doctor examined me in front of a group of resident ophthalmologists and, holding me in her hands, smiled at Savta and said, "He is such a nice baby – such a big head, a genius like Aristotle." Then turning to the doctors, she added, "Let's operate." One of the residents muttered, "I hope I won't be working that shift." After the meeting Savta sought him out and demanded to know what he had meant. "At this age his skull is so soft," he told her, "and this surgery would surely damage him." "We're planning to go to Israel in a few years," she told him. "Could we wait that long?" "Yes," he affirmed. "In fact, I think it would be much safer to have it done by a Jewish doctor." Realizing the implication that harm might come to her grand-

---

* "Savta" is the Hebrew word for "grandmother."

child, Savta packed our bag and immediately took the slow
train 1,000 miles back to Levov.

Over the next three years, I became aware of my blindness.
It was an uncomfortable, shadowy world – always dark.
Many sounds were sudden and unexpected. I seldom knew
where I was. The world was all hard surfaces and sharp
edges, and only Savta was soft and tender.

Only she could soothe and comfort me. The world seemed
a little brighter when she was near, and I clung to her, listened
for her, and followed her everywhere. When she went shopping or to the library, even though she assured me she was
coming right back, I would scream the entire time she was
away. My mother, of course, couldn't hear me, and even
when she saw I was having a tantrum, she couldn't stop me.
Only when Savta returned and I heard her sweet, loving
voice and felt her warm hug could I calm down.

When I was four, my family began the process of emigrating
to Israel. Although we lived comfortably in Levov, my father
was always in danger since his shop sold illegal photographs
of church icons, and my grandfather was too aware of the
dangers from the authorities. As Jews, my family felt it
would be better to live in a country governed by their own
people.

At that time, it was forbidden to emigrate directly from
Russia to the West, so we first had to cross the border into
Poland. We managed this, thanks to the paper Grandfather
had received when he was liberated from Siberia, stating that
he was born in Poland (and thanks also, I've been told, to a
bribable border guard). We had to stay there for six months
before we were permitted to leave.

In Poland I had my first eye operation for removal of
cataracts. It was excruciating and I couldn't understand what
was happening. Each night, Savta lay beside me, massaging
my neck and face. I remember waking up for a moment

during the operation and *seeing* a doctor's face – his surgical mask and his eyes. I don't know whether I was dreaming it or if I really did see him, but whatever happened, it was the first intimation that I might actually see, and that image and the hope it instilled never left me.

After the operation, both my eyes were completely covered with bandages. When they were removed, I was able to distinguish light, shadows, and even some vague shapes. People generally assume that blindness is submersion in total darkness, but after experiencing absolute blindness with the bandages on my eyes, I realized that blindness is relative and that I did have a little sight.

I recovered from the operation at home, and after six months in Poland, my grandparents, parents, two uncles, Bella, and I took our Polish passports and left for Italy, where we boarded the passenger ship *Shalom* and sailed to Israel.

I remember the crisp sea air and its salty spray, the big diesel engines which I not only heard but also felt through the deck, and the swaying of the ship which made it difficult for me to stand. And I remember the light – the brilliant silver sunlight which I could barely discern reflecting off the Mediterranean. I stood at the rail and stared at the light on the water for a long time. One time when I was there, my grandmother put a piece of cheddar cheese in my hand, and I remember holding it very close to my face and actually seeing my three fingers holding it, and seeing a marvelous color that I had never seen before. "That is yellow cheese, my darling Meir." Grandmother must have noticed my eyes trying to focus on the cheese. "Yellow cheese! Yellow cheese!" I shouted over and over, to whomever would listen, as I stumbled around the deck.

We landed in Haifa and settled in Morasha, a suburb of Tel Aviv. My grandparents and my uncles moved into one small apartment, and my family moved into another in the same building. Father and Grandfather set about re-establishing their photography business in Tel Aviv.

Over the next two years, I had four more cataract operations. A cataract is a progressive clouding of the lens. In successful cataract surgery, the lens is removed to allow light to penetrate to the retina. In my case, not only were the clouded lenses not completely removed, but the operations created scar tissue which further blocked the passage of light. My vision showed no improvement whatsoever.

These operations were terribly painful, and emotionally traumatic. I could hear children crying, doors slamming, and strangers speaking roughly. I was thirsty, and I hated the smells in the hospital. I was nearly always frightened. Savta was my only solace; she would hold me, soothe me, and massage me. We were in a hospital near Jaffa, on the Mediterranean, and she constantly reminded me to feel the refreshing sea breezes and smell the salty air. The one night I had to spend without her I cried the whole time.

After five operations, my lenses were almost totally destroyed. Without glasses I could see only blurred light and shadow, and with very thick glasses I could make out some vague shapes. Dr Stein, a world-famous ophthalmologist who performed this last operation, pronounced my condition irreversible, and I was certified as legally blind by the state of Israel. I was six years old.

At home, I was angry and rebellious. I would throw my glasses on the floor and stamp on them. The way they concentrated light on my eyes was painful, and although the lenses were too thick to break, I did succeed in wrecking the frames. I had persistent pain in my eyes, and I felt helplessly caught in a dark prison of shadows and outlines.

At the same time I was aware of a part of me that was peaceful, and accepted whatever happened. Even in my most hysterical moments, I knew that things were not as bad as they seemed.

I was always using my hands to "see" textures and shapes. I loved to feel my family's outlines – their faces, hands, arms, bellies, legs, and feet. Although my senses of smell, taste, and hearing were unusually acute, it was through touch that I really explored and came to know the world.

Since my world was not visual, communicating with my deaf parents was difficult. I did not learn sign language, and I never understood the importance of directing my lips to their eyes when I spoke. My father would grab my head, sometimes against my will, and pull my face upwards to read my lips. His voice sounded like a leaky faucet dripping into a coffee can – "Boop bop blip blue blue blob . . . ," but I developed an ear for understanding him, and knew when he was telling me to "Stop knocking over the damn lamp."

Of course there were many disasters. When my father and I went out together, I often got lost. I'd stand there and wail, but he couldn't hear me. I needed a Good Samaritan to figure out the problem and bring us together.

I always tried as hard as I could to be like others – I never accepted being "handicapped." When I crossed the street, I could see enough to know when the vague shapes of people began to move. Only when it was dark could I barely make out a red or green dot on the traffic light. Occasionally I'd just plow ahead, and drivers had to slam their brakes all around me. I was bumped several times, though not badly, and quite a fuss was made. But I never used a white cane or a guide dog.

I went to the movies, and although my eyes didn't tell me much, I could hear the plot. And I was never afraid of asking. I even rode a bicycle, though I often rode it into walls, trees, and people. Once I rode down a long set of stairs and banged my tailbone badly. I played soccer. Though I couldn't keep up with all the action, occasionally I got to kick the ball, and I was a good fighter. I loved to run around, but I fell down and bumped my head almost every day. Even today people say I have a hard head.

The kids in my neighborhood mostly excluded me. When I tried to join them, they played tricks on me. One minute they were there and the next minute they were gone. They saw nothing wrong with bullying me; it seemed perfectly natural to them. I had to shout and fight to join in any game and I had to work very hard to compete once I was in.

Finally I reached school age. We lived in the suburbs and the county provided transportation for all the handicapped children who had to attend schools in the city. In my van were one other blind boy and several kids with polio. Every morning and afternoon this group of blind and crippled children rode in and out of Tel Aviv.

I was fascinated by the city. It was so big and busy and noisy. I got to brag to the kids in my neighborhood about the big school I attended in the city. I could tell them about different games we played in Tel Aviv, and any time I lost a game, I would always say, "In Tel Aviv, we play by different rules."

In first grade, I started Braille class. The blind kids had an hour of instruction in reading and writing Braille at the end of each day. I found it difficult to sit in one place and concentrate on the raised impressions on the paper. The different arrangements of dots didn't make any sense to me. My first Braille teacher was a very impatient woman who yelled at me and punished me whenever I made a mistake, which made it difficult to learn.

In Braille class, when I wanted to look at my fingers passing along the text, my teacher yelled at me, "You can't see it anyway so don't look at it." This instruction to refrain from looking at my fingers, just to look straight ahead in order to fully concentrate on what the fingers felt, was especially annoying. It meant acting as though I had no eyes at all. By discouraging us from using what little sight we had, the teacher diminished the likelihood of our ever becoming "normal" and inadvertently helped lower our self-esteem.

There was another dilemma for handicapped kids. On the one hand, as a blind boy, I was not expected to accomplish very much. It was understood that reading and studying in Braille was slow and laborious. Yet, because of this, in order to compensate, I was also expected to work twice as hard as "normal" kids. This of course was very frustrating. Yet the more I was around "normal" kids, the more I realized I could do whatever they could and I was determined to. By the fourth grade, I was reading quite quickly in Braille.

When I was ten, we moved to Tel Aviv, and I had to learn my way around a whole new neighborhood. I continued at the same school since that was where Braille was taught, so I didn't get to meet the kids in my new neighborhood. I was quite lonely, and I took refuge in books. I read voraciously.

In Israel, there is intense competition to get into high school. My teachers never believed that a blind boy could get into a good high school, but my grandmother was determined to help me. She encouraged me to excel, tutored me as best she could with her broken Hebrew, and made sure that I believed in myself. I prepared intensively for high school, realizing that this would be a turning point in my life. With the help of my grandmother, who lobbied on my behalf with the principals of the top schools, I was accepted to the highest rated school in Tel Aviv.

Despite all my fears and doubts, I was exuberant about starting high school. The possibilities seemed limitless. This excitement was the excitement of the unknown. I had been encouraged, even pushed, to succeed by my grandmother and a few others who believed in me. But I immediately encountered the same narrow views about the handicapped as before. I was forbidden to go on field trips, and I was excluded from pre-military training, which was compulsory for all the other boys.

In Israel, military training is a basic part of every young person's life. To be excluded was quite a blow. I appealed to the assistant principal, telling him that I was perfectly capable of doing everything that was required. It took several hours – I even pounded on his desk – and he finally let me take the training and also the field trips. They wouldn't let me shoot a gun, but I could run as fast as anyone else. When the other boys had to jump ten feet down onto a mattress, I was not supposed to do it, but I sneaked into the group and jumped anyway. I was able to push myself into every part of the training except for rifle practice. The instructor was very firm about that. Here again I faced that unnerving contradiction. Because the instructor thought I didn't belong in the class in the first place, I had to do more than everyone else to justify being there. Although others could sometimes forget their uniforms, I always had to be dressed correctly. I didn't like being required to be anything more or less than everyone else.

I no longer had Braille instruction – this was a high school for normal children. Many of the required textbooks were not available in Braille, and although some of the teachers tried to help me by asking other kids to read to me, usually I had to write to the Braille library and request that the books be typed out in Braille for me. This, on top of many long, arduous hours of study, demanded that I adapt myself to completely new circumstances. I had to use my intelligence more fully and in different ways. I had to grasp ideas and facts very quickly; I couldn't simply read about them later like the other kids. Since I needed extra help with subjects like math, and also needed help with reading, I had to be very strong in other subjects so that I could exchange tutoring with other kids. I not only had to get by, I had to excel.

I did well in most of my classes, but I was failing my class in Talmud, Jewish law, because my teacher was more interested in soccer and the girls in my class than in giving a coherent lecture. I depended on the class lectures because the written material was not available to me. My Uncle Moshe, a well-known Biblical scholar who interpreted the Old Testament from a Marxist viewpoint, offered to tutor me. He felt that anything worth doing was worth doing perfectly. I would sit and read a page to him using two very thick magnifying glasses one on top of the other, and if I made even one small mistake, he would bend over and say caustically, "Pretty weak in this subject, eh?" It was difficult for him to sit patiently while I read so slowly, and it made me work all the harder to win his approval.

I also discovered girls that year, but at my first school dance, no girls would dance with me. Considering my great expectations for success in high school, this was a terrible disappointment.

In the summer following my first year in high school, at the suggestion of my regular ophthalmologist, I was examined by the head optometrist at the Hadassah Hospital in Jeru salem. She had a lot of sophisticated equipment to examine my eyes. After studying me carefully, she prescribed two types of magnifying lenses which, for the first time, would enable me to see letters. One lens was a monocle of telescopic strength with which I could read words on the blackboard, a letter or two at a time. The other was a cylindrical, micro-scopic lens which attached to the frame of my glasses and allowed me to read printed words, also a letter or two at a time. To read, I had to put the book right up to my nose.

It was scary. Of course I wanted to see, but I already knew how to function as a blind person, and it was frightening to think about changing that. Even though it was very difficult, I knew how to be blind and I was, in a manner of speaking, "comfortable" with that.

I was forced to confront the belief Braille teachers and others had instilled in me – that I couldn't use my eyes, and therefore shouldn't try. At 16, I had become so set in my ways, it was difficult and frightening to take the next step.

During the summer, I tried to adjust to the close-up lens by reading a short novel. It took me 45 hours to read 50 pages, but in spite of the great effort and the strain on my eyes and neck, I was exhilarated. When I began Braille, it had been just as slow, so I patiently waited for further improvement.

Sometimes I wonder how I managed to read or write at all – I had just learned what a letter looked like. During my second year of high school I did all the reading, wrote all the assigned papers and even passed the written tests. I did have agonizing headaches daily and often got nosebleeds from the strain. It was so difficult for me to write that I perspired heavily during tests. One teacher returned a bloodied paper to me saying, "You really put blood, sweat, and tears into this."

My math teacher treated me like an invalid and expected me to be quiet and self-effacing. He offered me more help than I needed. He even asked another student to take notes for me in class. I told him that after nine years of having to be helped with reading and writing, I wanted to do the work myself no matter how difficult.

Some of my classmates began to treat me as a peer, but many continued to harass me. Once when I needed help with a long geography assignment, I asked another student for help. He replied, "You have the book, read it." At first I resented this response, but after a while I realized the value of this lesson: I needed to be independent.

One day the Army Registration Department called. My father, whose deafness had kept him out of the Army, said that I should just show them my certificate of blindness, so I wouldn't have to go in for testing. This made me angry, because as I mentioned, serving in the Army is an important part of life in Israel, and I wanted nothing more than to be accepted. When I went to the Induction Center for my physical, the ophthalmologist was amazed when I couldn't read even the first letter on the Snellen chart – with my thick glasses on! I was declared ineligible to serve.

About that time, my ophthalmologist tested my progress with the magnifying lens. She knew I had been working hard, and complimented me, but after examining my strong right eye, she said, "Some kind of cataract is reappearing. I don't want to operate yet, but let's watch it closely and see what happens." I asked her, "Do you think my eyes can improve at all? Can any surgery improve them?" She answered, "No, I'm afraid not." I went home very depressed. Even if I were to take a chance on more surgery, there was no real possibility, according to the doctor, that it would improve my vision.

And yet, deep inside I had a different feeling. I was now able to see letters with a magnifying lens, and I knew that I would learn to read much faster. I *knew* the doctor must be wrong. I didn't know what improvements were possible, but I was convinced a solution would come.

Chapter 2

Isaac

Savta was having a difficult time. She helped Grandfather in the small shop where they sold my father's photographs. It was on a narrow alley near the Carmel Market in Tel Aviv, a noisy street with a few dingy restaurants – a bad location for such a business. The lack of business also discouraged my father so much that he lost interest in taking pictures.

Grandmother's escape was through books. Though her Hebrew was still rough, she was well-educated, and she read Russian novels endlessly. Her other delight was her grandson. Her love for me was something I can't possibly describe. Going to see her on Friday nights, celebrating the Sabbath together, being fed by her – I looked forward to it all week. The bread she sliced and buttered tasted so good to me that I thought it must be the most delicious food anyone had ever eaten. She would hug me and hold my arm, ask how things were with me, how I was getting along in school, what she could do for me. Though I couldn't make out her features, I knew there was a glow of tenderness around her. It was the most exquisite delight to be loved with every look, gesture, and thought.

Every week Savta would send me to a little lending library to exchange her books. I loved doing this for her. Miriam, the elderly woman who owned the library, always had a stack of books waiting for me. She sensed the love between

Savta and me. Miriam always sat me down in her chair and talked with me while she worked. I could hear the smile in her voice as she said, "I know you must be a good student. I'll bet you're really smart," in her strong Russian accent. She appreciated that I wasn't held back by being blind, and she especially liked seeing a blind boy coming for books. I felt like a courier carrying love between Miriam and Savta, and it was a joy for me.

Miriam took an interest in health and especially in massage and movement. She had recently helped a boy around my age named Isaac overcome severe near-sightedness by giving him a book of eye exercises. Miriam told my grandmother that Isaac could now read much faster and that I might benefit from meeting him.

When Grandmother told me about this, I wasn't too excited. I knew no one could help me read any faster, especially with my magnifying lens. But one day Isaac phoned me, and we arranged to meet at the library.

Miriam introduced us. Isaac impressed me as a very confident, sharp young man, though in fact he was only 16. He immediately asked me to take off my thick, dark glasses, and he looked at my eyes. After positively stating that my eyes could be cured, he asked who my doctor was. When I told him, he said, "She can't help you. She's very nice, and she means well and has a lot of experience; but she doesn't know anything about curing eye problems."

I was shocked. My first impulse was to run away. I thoroughly respected modern medicine, and I had never before questioned a doctor's knowledge or authority. Now this kid even younger than I was saying that my eyes could be cured and that my doctor knew nothing about curing eye problems! But as he continued to talk, I became more and more convinced that he was right.

I felt instinctively that Isaac was someone who might be able to help me. He promptly began describing all of my eye disorders. "Your eye muscles are very weak, which accounts

16

for your cross-eyedness, right? Your eyes look astigmatic, right? And you've been operated on more than once for cataracts, which has left you with scar tissue and floating membrane, right? Right!" "This is incredible," I told him. And he said, "I can show you some exercises that will improve your eyes."

A week later we met in Tel Aviv and stopped by my grandfather's shop to get money for busfare. Isaac studied him closely, and after we got on the bus, he told me in detail about Grandfather's heart problems, diabetes, and tendency for jaundice. I was amazed that he could know these things with just one glance. I later discovered that some people do have this faculty – to look at a person for the first time and not only pinpoint his or her problem, but also sense how to help. Later I discovered that I have a similar ability, but at the time it was all I could do to accept the notion that this was possible.

I asked Isaac whether he was a healer of some sort. I had heard about healers who seemed to have a magic touch or some incredible way of healing people. "No I'm not!" he snapped, "I help people heal themselves."

Isaac drew a diagram of my eye muscles and pointed to the weak or nonfunctioning ones. I looked at the diagram in a very strong light, but I could barely see the contrast of the white paper against the dark wooden table. I started to reach for my magnifying lens, but Isaac stopped me. "Stop relying on your glasses so much. Throw them away! I guarantee you'll be able to read without glasses in one year!"

The first exercise he showed me was one called "palming," a method for relaxing the eye muscles and nerves. I sat at a table with my elbows comfortably supported by a firm pillow and gently covered my closed eyes with my palms to prevent light from coming through. He told me to imagine something in motion. He said that he liked to sit in class and palm, and visualize someone digging a hole. I found it difficult to visualize something which I'd never seen. He also instructed me to visualize total blackness, and I had a hard time with that too.

Isaac learned these exercises from books Miriam had given him, all of which were accounts of the pioneering work of Dr William Bates. Dr Bates was an American ophthalmologist practicing at the turn of the century, who found through extensive and highly original research that the mind plays a major role in vision. According to Bates, physical or mental stress is the main cause of eye problems. When the eye relaxes, the correct cells of the eye are used, and vision is unimpaired. The key to Dr Bates's teaching is the correct usage of the eye, i.e. using the eye the way it works when it is relaxed. Accordingly, he developed and taught a whole system of exercises for the eyes which are designed to promote their correct function.

Ophthalmology has since discredited Bates' findings and his exercises. I think the main reason for this is that practicing the exercises takes time and discipline and patience, and not everyone is willing to give that much to improve their vision. But I would have given anything in the world to be able to see. I was ready to do anything Isaac told me to.

I felt exhilarated after my session with Isaac, and I ran to the bus and went straight home to tell my family about it. They were polite, but completely unable to understand or encourage me. I felt as though I were starting a new life, and I wanted everyone – my friends, family, teachers – to know. But only Isaac and Miriam could understand.

Isaac and I met again a week later, and this time he taught me "sunning," another important eye exercise created by Dr Bates which is done by facing the sun with *closed* eyes and turning the head gently from side to side. After I did this for a while, Isaac had me rest by palming, and then resume sunning. I asked him, "How do sunning and palming work?" "I don't want to tell you," he answered. "Just do it." I found this maddening. Still, from that time on I went up on to the roof of our apartment building several times a day to practice these exercises.

The following week, Isaac met me at our apartment. I was quite anxious, partly because he was coming to my home for the first time, but mostly because I was going to have my first date that evening. I had just bathed and dressed when he arrived, and he couldn't help noticing. "Hey, you look great," he said. This bolstered my confidence, and we went up to the roof so I could show him my sunning. Isaac watched briefly, then snapped at me, "Okay, stop it! Just sit down!"

I was startled, and he curtly explained that the idea was not to flail the head back and forth, but to turn it gently and slowly. He reminded me to alternate sunning with frequent periods of palming. After we settled down a little, Isaac began to encourage me to relax and enjoy the exercises, and not to strain myself while doing them. Then he sat silently for half an hour while I followed his instructions, and for the first time in my life, I knew what it was to relax. Though it was an unfamiliar feeling, it was wonderful, and it helped calm me for my date.

The session with Isaac turned out to be more satisfying than my first date. She was repelled by my thick glasses, and I must have bored her to tears with all my talk about sunning and palming. But it did help my self-esteem to finally have a date.

Once I began to do the exercises regularly and to really relax, I discovered how incredibly sensitive my eyes were to light. Even with closed eyelids, I could feel my eyes flinch from the sun, and when I covered them with my palms, brilliantly colored stars filled the darkness, sometimes for hours. This disturbed me so much that I telephoned Isaac. "Don't bother me about that. you're making too much of it," was all he had to say.

"All right," I replied, "I'll look it up in a book."

"You won't find your answer in any book," he laughed.

"It's really very simple, so simple it's a joke! But you'll have to find out for yourself!" And he hung up the phone. I was frustrated to the point of tears, but there was nothing I could do. This was just Isaac's way.

I continued sunning and palming faithfully every day. I spent nearly all my free time up on the roof. Sunning became more than just an eye exercise for me, it was my life.

During our next session Isaac taught me how to use blinking as an exercise. Dr Bates discovered that opening and shutting the eyelids frequently in a relaxed way releases tension in the eyes, preventing squinting, keeping the eyes moist, and increasing blood flow to the eyes. This is the natural way for the eyes to function. When he showed me this I realized how much tension I had in my eyes.

Early in the summer, Isaac took me to the beach to practice sunning, palming, and blinking, and to show me several stretches for my body. I enjoyed this so much that for the rest of the summer, I went to the beach as often as I could.

In mid-June, when the sun was highest in the sky, I especially enjoyed sunning and the other eye exercises. After sunning a lot, I would sit and palm for hours. At first, my chronic headaches and eye pains just seemed to be getting worse. But this was caused by the relaxation exercises, which allowed my body to finally feel all the years of accumulated tension. Realizing this, I continued the eye exercises and stretches even more religiously, and by August the pain began to subside. This was encouraging, and my enthusiasm for exercising increased even more.

There were times my headaches were so severe I couldn't move. One evening at my Grandmother's house, I sat down in front of the television, and as I strained my eyes to see, my headache became unbearable. My Uncle Zvi, who lived with Savta, sat down next to me and started rubbing my temples. It was painful, but he assured me that massage could help dissolve a headache. And the headache did decrease.

Though Zvi knew nothing about massage, he knew instinctively what needed to be done.

Once I learned that massaging the temples and scalp could relieve headaches, I began doing it myself. I discovered that after massaging my temples and improving the circulation to my eyes, the outlines and shapes were a little less fuzzy, a little more distinct.

I had my first crush that summer. I couldn't see my "heart-throb," but I imagined her to be very beautiful (although I had no idea what that meant). My crush was completely a fantasy, but one thing was sure – I was becoming very aware of girls, their sound and smell and shape and touch. Whatever good-looking was, everyone seemed to agree that certain girls were and that I wasn't.

When I was a child, the other kids called me "monkey," which in Hebrew has the connotation of extreme ugliness. I believed them, and today when I look at pictures from that time, I can see that I did look something like a monkey. But Savta always thought I was fine-looking, and I believed her more than the kids. I used to press my nose against the mirror and yell, "I am not a monkey! I'm gorgeous!" But when it came to a possible relationship with a girl, I felt like a monkey again.

Now for the first time I began to experience some self-confidence and hope of overcoming my handicap. But, as my vision began to improve, I became reluctant to use my sense of touch, and I began to bump into walls and people again, falling down stairs, and stumbling off the curb into the street.

Only Miriam seemed to understand the problems of this transition, and she encouraged me to use my sense of touch more. She also taught me some basic massage. Miriam never told me very much about herself and her training, but she did share a few stories. From the age of seven, she had many ailments, and she found that movement was very helpful in

21

overcoming them. She had two paralyzed toes and very flat feet, and a famous orthopedist prescribed a heavy boot and told her that her condition would progressively degenerate. She was thoroughly convinced his advice was not correct; she cried for all the people he was "helping." Instead of following his prescription, she went home and did exercises in her bathtub, moving her toes in circles under the water. She walked every day and went on long hikes every week, and so managed to overcome the paralysis.

Miriam suffered from chronic rapid, irregular heartbeat. A movement education teacher showed her how to move various parts of her body while he massaged her chest around the heart, and that not only regulated her heartbeat but taught her the subtle connections between different parts of the body.

After Miriam delivered her first child, she suffered a prolapse of the uterus. She told her doctor that in two months she would have it back to normal. In fact it took only a month of intensive pelvic exercises for her to move the uterus back in place.

Miriam made it clear that her deep understanding of the body was based more on intuition and experience than on technical knowledge. She respected the knowledge of doctors but often questioned the way they used that knowledge. She had a very strong intuitive sense of movement, and loved to experiment with it, exploring all the different ways there are to move the body. And she loved to share her knowledge.

I had been rubbing my temples, but until Miriam showed me, I had never thought to massage my eyebrows, eyelids, eyelashes, and all of the bones, muscles, and skin surrounding my eyes. As I massaged away the pain of the headaches, they were replaced by a burning sensation in my eyes. My eyes were beginning to feel the accumulated fatigue from years of squinting and staring. Straining to see kept me from blinking enough. Isaac explained to me the importance of blinking to rest, massage, and moisten the eyes.

22

I started eleventh grade with a confident, relaxed feeling about the future. The horizons I had imagined when I entered high school paled in comparison to what I now envisioned. Six months previously Isaac had said that within a year I would be seeing well, and I was determined to realize that.

After months of fanatically sunning, palming, and blinking, Isaac taught me shifting, an exercise to improve visual acuity, and in my case to control my still-horrendous nystagmus. Nystagmus is an involuntary flutter of the eyes which can severely impair seeing. Shifting helped me learn to focus on specific objects and introduced me to "conscious vision," that is, seeing with your mind as much as with your eyes. With or without glasses, I could only see one big blur, so Isaac instructed me to look for details. For example, he said that when I looked at buildings, I should try to make out the position of the windows. He meant that when I looked, I should assume that the building had windows, and then try to locate them. There was a tall building which I passed on my way to the beach, not far from where I lived. I stood there every day for several weeks trying to relax my eyes so the nystagmus would slow down and images appear. I imagined what windows might look like and tried to find them somewhere I supposed they might be. And finally, one Friday night, I *saw* them. I phoned Isaac to announce my triumph but he was unimpressed. He told me, "Now look for the air conditioners. They're in the lower parts of the windows." Of course I had never seen an air conditioner, and I couldn't guess what one might look like. But I practiced shifting for hours every day, and after only a week I was able to make out what I thought must be the air conditioners.

In this way, I slowly began to educate my eyes to see. Until then I had seen the world only as a single blurred unit. Now I was learning to divide that entity into details. By developing the habit of looking for specific things where they should be, I gradually activated my eyes and brain for the process of seeing. For 16 years, I had been learning not to look, not to see, not to try to find anything. Everyone else would always find things for me. No one, not even I, ever expected me to see. But now my eyes were full of windows and air conditioners, and my brain was beginning to function differently.

After six months of eye exercises, I no longer needed the cylindrical magnifying lens, only a pair of glasses. My astonished optometrist had to cut my prescription in half. Without glasses, I could see shapes, light and dark, and a little movement. With glasses, I was now seeing windows and air conditioners, the girls in my class, and even my own face in the mirror. I could make out the contrast between the color of my hair and my skin; and I could see my nose, my lips and ears, and even a pimple on my chin! Six months earlier, I could not see my face, and now when I looked really carefully, I could even see my eyes.

It was hard for my family to accept my improvement. I knew my vision was getting better, but they still regarded me as blind, especially since my "doctor" was a teenager, and my therapy some "meaningless movements." They tried to get me to stop doing eye exercises. This unorthodox approach seemed to threaten everything they believed in. How the exercises worked and what I was trying to accomplish were of no interest to them. Just as my Braille teachers expected me to accept my fate and learn to live with it, my family was afraid my expectations were unrealistically high and I would just be disappointed later.

My grandfather was especially hard on me. He loved to be sick himself so he could be the center of attention. He had every symptom in the book, though the causes were vague. He called them "attacks." Treating me as an invalid seemed to make him feel better. He would tell me not to carry heavy packages, play rough games, get into fights, or do practically anything the least bit dangerous. When I couldn't find something, he delighted in showing me where it was and how easy it had been to find it. "You're as blind as ever," he taunted me. "Your exercises are doing no good at all!"

Grandfather hated the fact that I was turning my back on "real" physicians. "This kid Isaac is even younger than you are," he scoffed. "Are you trying to tell me a 16-year-old dropout can cure your blindness?"

I had hoped that my great-uncle Moshe would be more understanding. He had made so much effort to help me with reading, and he had always struggled for recognition for his own unconventional ideas. But he also couldn't understand how a boy of 16 could be of any help for me, and he couldn't give me much support either. Uncle Moshe had contracted throat cancer at the age of eighty. I visited him regularly at the hospital. One day when I came into his room, he was asleep. I sat quietly and watched him with my limited vision. It looked as if a smile was forming on his face, and it seemed to me his breathing was becoming deep and regular. At that moment I was able to see my uncle as if he were bathed in light. I could distinguish his closed eyes, the grey stubble of his beard, even the gentle rising and falling of his abdomen as he breathed. I must have sat there for half an hour as my vision grew brighter and brighter. I saw an old man near death who could dream about his life with satisfaction. Then he began to wake up to the reality of his hospital room and his pain. The smile left his face and I again had trouble seeing him. We talked quietly for awhile, and I left.

The following day, Isaac was disturbed about something and needed to talk with me. This was rare, so I stayed and listened, and I missed seeing my uncle. His wife phoned me and angrily demanded why I had missed going to the hospital. The next day when I went to see Uncle Moshe he too was upset, and he began to bait me. "Why is this Isaac helping you for nothing? He must be a homosexual on the make." I couldn't believe he said that. I was so disturbed I ran all the way home and threw myself on to my bed, sobbing. It seemed no one could see Isaac for his true worth.

My mother came into my room and stroked my hair, soothing me. She was the first to see the improvement in my eyes, and although she had not trusted Isaac initially, she always thought he was a good kid. Mother's support at that moment was crucial. It was almost unbearable trying to convince the rest of my family that the work on my eyes was of value.

I continued visiting Uncle Moshe in the hospital, and I knew he was dying. We sat together for hours on end, talking about his ideas, and mine. He never complained about his pain, and I found this inspiring. His spiritual strength and toughness kept him removed from the pain and from the sordid aspects of dying. He seemed to be living in another realm of consciousness.

The dreadful last days finally came. One morning Aunt Esther phoned to tell me Uncle Moshe was dead. I couldn't say a thing, but after the funeral, in spite of my grief, I felt a great peacefulness. While everyone else mourned, I felt like smiling. I knew my uncle had not really died – only his body had given out. I felt that this was a wonderful secret that no one could share with me. His strong affirmation of life is still with me, and to this day I can still see him sleeping in the hospital with that peaceful, radiant smile.

Soon after, at my eye doctor's request, I went to Jerusalem to have my eyes tested again. While there, I visited my Uncle Sadi, a prestigious engineer, and his younger brother, my Uncle Zvi, who was also visiting. At dinner, my Aunt Nayima, Sadi's wife, questioned me about Isaac. I explained how Isaac supported himself, and many other details about him. Their questioning became more and more hostile, and only Uncle Zvi's girlfriend came to my defense. "What do you all want from Meir anyway? Why are you all so against what he's doing? I think it sounds great. If you won't encourage him, then why don't you at least leave him alone." This led to an enormous family row. They told her to shut up and said that I was an idiot and a sucker. I was devastated. What a way to talk to a young man burning with zeal for a new way of life!

Uncle Sadi had the last word. "Look, kid, I changed your diapers and wiped your ass – so listen to me!" Then he drew what he thought was a picture of the eye and explained that in my case the pupils were missing and that I would never be able to see normally. He had no idea that the pupil is simply an empty space in the middle of the eye. My eyes were then so sensitive to light that the pupils were always contracted almost to a pinpoint. But my uncle just *knew* that there was something irreversibly wrong with my eyes and that I should forget about ever seeing normally.

This was an unhappy time for me. Isaac happened to be in Jerusalem at the same time and took me to the hospital for my examination. He knew I was upset because my nystagmus, which had been improving, was worse again. Nystagmus reacts immediately to stress. Because of this, I tested badly, and the optometrist decreased the lens prescription by only a little. When I told my uncle about the improvement, he said, "Is that all? Well, you're still legally blind."

"Maybe I should give up trying to convince anyone," I thought. "People don't want to accept the truth of my eyes improving, even when it's right in front of them." But I knew it was very important for me to convince others, especially my family, and I realized that the only way to convince anyone would be to show them.

Soon after returning from Jerusalem, I went to visit my grandparents. Grandfather was in bed with one of his "attacks." His hands and feet were icy cold. I had been practicing some of Miriam's massage techniques on myself, so I took his right hand and massaged it gently, moving all the joints to relieve their stiffness. I felt something like tiny granules under the skin of his palms and fingers, so I massaged them until they disappeared. Gradually the color returned to his skin – which I could see! – and he began to feel warmth in both hands and both feet, even though I had only worked on one hand. "What are you, some kind of magician?" he laughed nervously.

"But see how much better you feel?" Savta pointed out.

"Okay, so it's better. But he is acting like a magician."

At our next session a few weeks later, Isaac looked closely at my eyes and said, "I don't think you need the cylinder anymore." Soon after that my eyes were tested by a doctor, and she confirmed that I no longer needed it, saying "This is impossible. No astigmatism is correctable." But in fact, I could read better without the cylinder, so she lowered my prescription, and told me that after the next reduction I would no longer be legally blind.

Isaac said I should read only with these new glasses. It was difficult to adjust to reading without the cylinder. In the beginning, it took me four hours to read one page. I needed very strong light, and even then I sometimes missed letters or even whole words. My mind wandered. It was difficult to concentrate for that long, and it was an enormous strain on the rest of my body. One time I tried so hard to read a single page that I suddenly threw up. "It takes so much time," I complained to Isaac. "So use your spare time," he shrugged.

He watched me read. "You are missing words." Then he showed me an exercise to help me shift my eyes and move my focus from point to point, so that I wouldn't miss details. He explained that shifting the focus in this way enables you to make use of the macula, the part of the eye that sees the most clearly but can only take in one small detail at a time. By learning to focus on small details and developing the habit of seeing each detail clearly and separately, I could make use of the macula, and my vision steadily improved.

One day I was playing soccer at school and got some dust in my eyes. It was extremely irritating, and I went to the school nurse to have my eyes washed out. But she just administered eye drops and suggested I continue using them at home. After several days my eyes started burning so badly that I had to stay home from school. Sunning didn't help; in fact it aggravated the condition. I closed myself up in a completely dark room and I lay down and palmed, with a towel over my face and hands, while I listened to rock and roll. The music kept me company, and the palming and darkness helped to relax my eyes and bring moisture to them. I was sure I was doing exactly the right thing. Then I began to blink, faster than I ever had before. At first my eyes grew more moist because of the resting and palming I'd been doing, but then they became dry again. Something drove me to continue blinking for a very long time, probably more than an hour. Eventually the itchy dryness went away, and my eyes began to tear profusely, washing away not only the dust particles but also the eye drops.

I continued to blink, covering my eyes gently with my palms, and the tears continued to flow as if I were crying. It was utterly amazing. I palmed for two more hours, and then tried sunning again. This time the sun did not disturb me, and my eyes no longer burned. From then on my eyes have been considerably less sensitive to light and better able to protect themselves from dust and weather. The sunning probably helped a little, but I believe it was the fast blinking and the palming in a darkened room for several hours which produced those remarkable results. Isaac had been telling me that I didn't blink enough, and from that day on I began to blink a lot, so much that people stared at me. The fact that I was able to recognize and respond to my body's needs clearly indicated how much my eyes were improving.

.

Chapter 3

Miriam

One Sunday evening Miriam invited me to her house for dessert. Over tea and chocolate cake I told her about Isaac's prediction that I would be able to see perfectly in one year. She answered, "Even if you don't, even if you still have to wear glasses, it's far better to be using your eyes correctly than to go on using them wrong, to have eyes that are becoming more alive with movement and not just staring." She asked me about my eye exercises and then she asked, "Do you work on the rest of your body also?" "Sometimes," I answered. "The calf muscles are connected to vision, you know," she said. Although my own calves were thin and my ankles and feet tense and contracted, I was taken aback when she connected this to vision.

As Miriam explained more, she became quite excited. For 56 years she'd been exercising, always trying to help her body feel better. Every day she discovered something new. Her enthusiasm was contagious, and I immediately recognized that I too wanted to try this movement therapy she was telling me about. "Why do we need movement," I asked her, "and what is the correct way to move?"

"We need movement because that is what life is about," she replied. "There is no such thing as a completely sick person, or a completely healthy person either, for that matter. There are only those who move more and those who move less. Movement in the human body is continuous. Once it stops we stop living. There is either restriction to movement or freedom of movement, and a person can choose either. The correct motion is circular, rotating, and fluid, not angular or jerky. The round movements are beneficial because the basic cell structure is round and our muscles want to move that way." She continued, her Russian accent thickening as she became more and more animated, "The human body has 600 muscles, but the average person uses only around 50. Our potential is so enormous! We could use so many more muscles than we do!" I was in awe. I had never thought about this before.

Miriam began to show me some exercises. We stood up and moved our heels up and down, keeping our toes on the ground. Then we kept our heels on the ground and moved our toes up and down. We got down on all fours and moved our shoulders in a circular motion. We stood leaning with our hands against the wall and our elbows straight, shifting pressure from one wrist to the other to stretch our shoulders. Finally we simply rotated our heads. After that, my back felt much straighter and my head higher. After finishing dessert and talking for another hour, Miriam announced, "Meir, I expect you to be teaching me in two months time."

I went home, and even though I was too excited to practice the exercises that night, the next night and every night from then on I sat for twenty minutes before bed, stretching my neck and rotating my head. I discovered that if I did this stretch before reading, the words on the page appeared clearer. I also did the shoulder exercises that Miriam had demonstrated, and my shoulders felt looser and stronger.

Every day after school, I closed the door to my room and exercised for an hour – first some stretching exercises that Isaac had taught me, and then the exercises Miriam and I had done. I also ran in place, lifting my knees high and dropping my feet heavily to shake the tension from my foot muscles.

31

Within a month my thigh muscles had built up noticeably, and new muscles began to appear in my calves.

When Miriam saw me, the change in my posture was obvious, and when I demonstrated some of the new exercises I had discovered, she said, "I knew you would be teaching me." This time Miriam taught me the importance of breathing. "You must always breathe through the nose, like in yoga. Your breathing should be deep and comfortable, always directed to your abdomen." She suggested that I go to the beach and do my eye exercises standing in shallow water; the movement of the waves would stimulate my foot and calf muscles. A new world was opening up for me. By the end of the session I felt that I was receiving a precious gift of valuable knowledge about the body.

These "anti-calisthenic" movements were not just exercises, they reflected an extraordinary attitude about the body. Rotating motions involve more muscles, and in a more balanced way, than vertical or lateral motions. Miriam always tried to activate as many muscles as possible. She realized intuitively that many physical problems are due to a lack of movement, and can be relieved by learning proper movement. She particularly emphasized the importance of correct breathing. She believed that a lack of oxygen leads to disease.

With Miriam's guidance, I began to devote myself fully to the practice and study of movement, breathing, coordination, and the gentle rhythms of the body. Whenever I could, in summer or winter, I would go to the beach and stand in shallow water with the waves washing over my feet, lifting each foot in turn, and moving my head from side to side. It was pure bliss.

Once when I was standing in the water with my eyes closed, an old man nearby shouted, "What are you doing?" I was taken aback and embarrassed, but I answered, "Eye exercises." "Oh, eye exercises," he said. "I can show you yoga exercises that are much better. C'mon."

I was about to reply that there was nothing better for my eyes than what I was doing, but he was already twenty yards away, so I followed him onto the beach to see what he would show me.

The old man's face was brown and wrinkled, and what little hair he had was white. But his body looked very strong – many years younger than his face. "My name is Shlomo," he said, and he showed me an exercise which I liked immediately. It was very gentle. With my left hand I held the back of my head and moved it from side to side, while my right hand pressed firmly against my forehead. This exercise loosened my neck and massaged my forehead at the same time, which was very stimulating for my eyes. After just this one exercise, Shlomo excused himself, but told me to look for him, that he came to the beach every day.

The next day I found him leading a group of older men and women in exercises. When someone had a problem, he would correct it. His yoga stretches seemed unusual to me at first, but I came to see that they were actually simple and reflected his clear understanding of the body. I was quite weak and stiff, and found them difficult to do, but I could see the sense of them and I joined in gradually.

That afternoon I saw Miriam and asked her what she thought about yoga. "It's okay," she replied, "as long as you don't do it mechanically or passively. If you can do it actively and with awareness, it is wonderful."

The next morning, Shlomo told me, "You know there's no trick to it, no secret, there's not even any strenuous effort. It's simply a matter of moving every part of the body, from the tips of the toes to the crown of your head." This was exactly what Miriam had said!

Shlomo showed me a number of exercises which he found suitable for his body. He said his back was slightly stiff, but that he could barely bend it at all before he began exercising. He'd always had a tendency toward aches and pains, because his spinal disks had deteriorated from hard, physical labor as an Israeli pioneer. Yet he now appeared to have the strength and flexibility of a thirty-year-old! He could move each vertebra separately as he bent over.

Shlomo was pleased by my interest in his work, and he showed me many exercises. He moved his arms in circles, first the entire arm and then just the forearm. He clasped his hands with one arm behind his head and the other behind his back. While clasping his hands, he bent his upper body forward and rotated his spine. Then he lay stretched out on one side, and leaning his head on his hand in what he called "The Philisopher's Position," brought one knee to his forehead, and then bent that leg backward and touched the back of his head with his foot. Lying on his back he lifted one knee to his chest and then lifted his head with his hand to touch the knee to his forehead.

This old man's flexibility was very impressive! He told me he did many other exercises every day, and that one must do an exercise twenty or more times consecutively for it to really activate the joints and muscles.

Shlomo and I spent most of that summer together, stretching and doing yoga. One day he took me to a class in Tel Aviv given by Moshe Feldenkrais, a pioneer in the field of therapeutic movement. I learned some valuable things. Like Miriam, Feldenkrais recognized that any movement should take into account the whole body, and that the most effective movement is not strenuous, but is gentle.

Shlomo made a great contribution to the foundation of my ideas about exercise and bodywork. I was only seventeen and he was seventy-seven and I learned so much from him. His flexibility and innate sense of movement made a deep impression on me.

What a wonderful summer, climaxing the most important year of my 1ife! First Isaac taught me eye exercises and told me I would see without glasses. Then Miriam taught me gentle movement and breathing. And now Shlomo showed me stretches to loosen and strengthen my body even more. I knew I was at a crossroads.

Chapter 4

Danny

One autumn day during my last year of high school, while I was practicing sunning exercises after lunch, a classmate came over and asked what I was doing. David had been one of the few students who showed a positive interest in my work, and he had always been pleasant to me. A few times he'd even asked for my advice about some health problems.

David told me that his girlfriend, Adina, the prettiest girl in our class, was having such severe headaches that she was hardly able to sleep, and was also having frequent nightmares and irrational fears. I recommended that he talk with Isaac, and I helped arrange a meeting. David and Adina came to my house for a very successful session with Isaac. At the end, Adina said to me, "Thank you for helping me, Meir." I said, "The only thanks I want is for you to work on yourself." I was really happy to help, even if only indirectly.

But a few days later, Isaac disappeared for what turned out to be months. On the best of occasions, he was only available when he felt like it, but now he was completely abandoning both Adina and me. During all this time I felt I really needed guidance and direction. However, Isaac wasn't around, or if he was he wouldn't answer the phone when I tried to reach him. In spite of my concern and my hurt feelings, his influence and example remained strong. I continued to feel as if he was guiding my efforts.

Sometimes I would go down to Allenby Street, where all the felafel stands were, and have a felafel. It would remind me of Isaac, because he was crazy about felafel. Along one side of the street there was a row of felafel shops, each run by a different family, who made their felafel according to closely guarded secret recipes, mixing garbanzo flour with spices, oil and other ingredients, then shaping it into patties and frying it. The felafel was then stuffed into pita bread with vegetables and sesame butter, and you could either take it out or eat it there at small tables. There were always long lines at each booth. I had no special craving for felafel, but it made me feel connected to Isaac somehow.

It reminded me of the long hours we used to spend there, usually accompanied by some girl that he had brought along, talking about all kinds of things. Although it wouldn't actually occupy much of the conversation, it seemed to me that we were always talking either about my eyes or about health in general, subjects in which I was most interested, of course. I drank in everything he said with a tremendous thirst, and struggled to read his expression to understand the meaning behind his words. The things he had to say were of great importance to me, and had enormous influence on me. I remember him saying, "Every disease is curable. Your eye problems, Meir, can definitely be cured, in spite of all the operations and the thick glasses you've worn all your life. Your eyes will soon be cured and you will see perfectly."

I was particularly upset about Isaac's treatment of Adina, for I felt that he should have continued to see her at least until she showed some improvement. One day I went to Miriam's library, and Adina happened to be there. She seemed pleased to see me. Her condition was apparently getting worse, and she'd been in a lot of pain. Miriam overheard us and offered to show her some exercises, but before she did, she said, "Why doesn't Meir show you some exercises that he knows?" Adina was immediately interested, but I was hesitant. I finally allowed myself to be persuaded to see her at her home the following week. After she left, Miriam told me, "I won't work with you any more unless you work with Adina."

Every day that week, I went to the library to learn some exercises from Miriam which could help alleviate Adina's headaches. Then I went home and tried them out. Finally I went to Adina's house and taught her several that I thought would be especially good for her. She began doing them faithfully, and I returned once a week to work with her. After only a month of this, her headaches diminished considerably.

During my sessions with Adina, I learned that she was taking anti-depressant drugs prescribed by a psychiatrist. I told her I was afraid that the drugs might hurt her and I thought she should stop taking them. When she said this to her parents, they were enraged at me.

Miriam had the greatest respect for parents and would never do anything against their wishes. The day after this incident, Miriam suddenly announced that she was not going to be available to help either Adina or me. She said there were two reasons. "First, I'm working too hard already. The second reason I can't tell you. You'll have to figure it out for yourself."

First no Isaac, and now, no Miriam. I was stunned! What could I tell Adina? She had been doing her exercises with such eagerness and had placed so much trust in Miriam and me. I saw Adina in school the next day and tried to make something up, but the truth poured out. Adina was shocked, and nearly speechless. "But Miriam promised!"

Adina was on my mind all day. As I was doing my exercises at home in the afternoon, I concentrated on her head and shoulder tension and I began to feel as if my body became hers, experiencing her tension from within. I lay face down on the floor and lifted my upper body up and rotated my head and shoulders. This released a lot of tension and made that area feel looser and stronger. This was a new exercise for me, and I was sure it would be good for Adina. I devoted the rest of the afternoon to finding exercises for her.

I showed them to Adina the next day with an apology. "I'm not very good at this." "Don't say that," she protested. "I think you're as good as Isaac and Miriam. In fact, better – you're still here. You have a talent, Meir, and I trust you." Adina was my first student, and this compliment was a big encouragement for me.

Over the next few months, Adina's headaches and insomnia disappeared completely. I felt a tremendous sense of achievement. Adina had helped me believe in myself. She reaffirmed what I felt inside, and this was deeply satisfying.

One day, four months since I'd seen him, I bumped unexpectedly into Isaac. In fact, I didn't see him as we passed on the sidewalk. He saw me. Isaac slapped me on the back and said, "Still not talking to me, eh?" as if *I'd* abandoned *him*. But I was too glad to hear his voice to be angry.

We talked as he waited for the bus, and he told me, "You know, Meir, I feel that my work with you was important, not just because of what it will do for you, but because I know you will help other people. You have a very good instinct and your sense of touch is already better developed than some people with 20 years of experience. I expect you to become a great teacher."

I went home filled with inspiration. This brief encounter changed my life. I had dreamed of becoming a diplomat, or maybe a foreign minister. But when Isaac suggested healing, I knew he was right. His confidence awakened in me an awareness that had been dormant, that the work I was doing could become my life's work.

The same week that Miriam severed my dependence on her, she also stopped working on my friend Nayima, a polio victim who had had thirteen operations on her legs. Miriam met her when she was about to have her fourteenth operation, and convinced her to try exercising instead. She had introduced Nayima to me, so that we could encourage and learn from one another. Though our problems were different, we felt a strong bond, working together on "incurable" disabilities. We had to conquer our negative attitudes and then the problems themselves. We needed to decide not to be cripples.

Nayima had excruciating pains in both legs. The operations had caused a lot of damage. At Miriam's suggestion, Nayima worked on herself for two hours a day, and sometimes went on for another three or four hours after that. She did Miriam's exercises as well as some she found in books and some she invented herself. Nayima wanted to become a physical therapist, but her parents found this unsuitable for a proper Orthodox, Jewish woman and wanted her to marry and settle down. This was frustrating for her, and I listened to and supported her.

In spite of the pain, she loved walking, and we often walked together. One day we walked quite a distance to pick up a new pair of specially designed orthopedic shoes. She limped a little on the way home, but her walking wasn't too bad. At home, she said, "It's not my muscles that kept me going. They're too tired. It was just will power. This is farther than I've ever walked before." Nayima didn't just want to stop using a cane. She didn't even just want to climb mountains. She wanted there to be no difference between the way she walked and the way other people walked and she would do whatever she had to do to achieve this.

A young man named Eli, who was severely crippled with muscular dystrophy, was getting a lot of publicity in Israel at the time. He was trying to get accepted into the Army to show that someone severely handicapped could make a contribution to his country. He argued that he could serve Israel with his intelligence, even though his body was paralyzed. I supported his cause, but it was Nayima who thought to phone him and offer help.

Nayima told him that he was fighting too much against society and not enough against his muscular dystrophy. Eli responded that there was nothing he could do about the disease, and that he was in good shape compared to many others with his kind of muscular dystrophy. Nayima insisted, "There is a lot you can do about your disease, if you want to." I also spoke to him and managed to interest him in the possibility that we might be able to help him.

A few days later we went to his house in Tel Aviv. Eli had a handsome and sensitive face, but his body was the most deformed that either Nayima or I had ever seen. His head flopped on to one of his shoulders, and many of his bones were out of place.

"Are you shocked by the way I look?" he asked.

"No, I'm not," I answered, and I wasn't. I was too busy thinking about what we could do to help him.

Eli told us, "When I was born, the doctors said I wouldn't live three years. My vertebrae are totally out of alignment – they curve both left and right. My ribs are completely twisted around, and this shoves my heart over by my right armpit. It's funny when these famous doctors examine me with their stethoscopes and can't even find my heart!" He said that his body temperature was high and his palms and the soles of his feet were usually sweaty. He suspected that this warmth is what had kept him alive. I started to explain our work to him. "Rotating motions help all the muscles involved in the movement to work together, and to work and rest alternately. We can activate all of your muscles." Then Nayima told him about the benefits of massage for strained, tight, weak, or injured muscles. "The most important thing is to adjust the touch for your body." Eli told us that although he'd had physical therapy and hydrotherapy, only his back had ever been massaged. Nayima insisted that his whole body needed massage, and Eli promptly assented. When Nayima and I left Eli's house we were in complete agreement. Nayima felt that she, of the two of us, knew best how to work on his body, and she hinted at this several times. I didn't mind;

in fact I was happy to work with someone who felt so knowledgeable and confident.

A week later, Nayima and I went to Eli's house together. She had asked Miriam for advice on how to work with Eli, but after a short time she took off on her own. "Now the world has the Nayima Method," Eli joked.

His arms and legs were very crooked, and he couldn't straighten them out by himself. His muscles were thin and his hands were so weak that his skinny fingers curled up on to his palms. His ribs were completely misshapen, bulging out in some places and caving in in others. It was curious that I could see him so well. It was probably due to my great interest.

After only two sessions, Eli was able to hold his head fairly straight for about ten minutes and could move heavy books around on his desk. Even the muscles of his fingers and upper arms showed a little more substance.

After that Nayima and I began to work on him at different times, and we also trained the members of his adoptive family to work on him. Eli's improvement, though slight, was a great encouragement to me.

Then suddenly, out of the blue, Nayima told me, "Eli and I are going to get married." I could not believe my ears. It was not Eli's crippled condition that disturbed me, but the fact that Nayima was just eighteen, and they were deciding to marry after an acquaintance of just four weeks. I burst out laughing and said, "You're joking." But they weren't. I was stunned and skeptical, but my reaction was mild compared to the others they encountered. Her parents were frankly horrified at the idea, and refused even to listen to her. They were extremely religious people, and had not even imagined that Nayima would be allowed to choose her own husband – let alone to make the choice she had! Even Miriam was appalled, "Doesn't she know he's going to die in a couple of years? What kind of marriage will that be?" But the marriage never took place. Nayima's parents managed to stop it. The matter was finally decided by her Rabbi, who found her a Rabbinical student from New York City. Despite her rebellion against her parents, Nayima could not go against the Rabbi's wishes; he was the very spirit of her religion. For three sleepless nights, she agonized over the decision, and she finally decided not to marry Eli.

Eli was very despondent, but after a while he recovered from all of this, and I began working on him by himself. It was encouraging to see him get stronger. After only two months, he could hold his head up for an hour. I knew that he could be helped and that within five years he would be able to walk if he would work on himself.

Unfortunately, Eli's emotional roller coaster continued. Just four months after recovering from Nayima, he announced his plans to marry Tsippi, his adoptive sister. Their adoptive mother gave them two hours to pack and leave. They stayed at my house for a week until they found a place to live. Three days before the wedding, Tsippi's real mother came to their apartment to try to kill Eli, shouting that her daughter would not marry such a cripple. The police put her in custody and she remained in jail until after the marriage.

It wasn't long before Eli lost interest in my treatment. When I came to work on him, it was apparent that he hadn't exercised between my visits. Although his body had improved remarkably in a short time, he wasn't willing to go beyond that point. When he stopped working on himself, I had to accept this decision. I could only assist him, I couldn't magically heal him.

I continued to progress with my eyes. My goal was to be able to read without glasses, and I spent hours each day working towards this. I had stopped using the magnifying cylinder some months before and was reading with my new glasses. It took nearly four hours to read a page, which

I could read in ten minutes with the cylinder, but I was determined.

Sometimes my eyes grew very tired trying to read, so I would take my glasses off and put my nose right down on to the page, and to my astonishment, sometimes the letters would appear. Then I would try to guess what the word containing those letters might be, and to my amazement, there would be the whole word. But I remembered that Isaac had told me to read only with the glasses, so I put them back on. At times I even took my grandmother's glasses, which had a much weaker prescription, and read for a while with them. But I found the challenge of reading without glasses irresistible, and I tried it more and more frequently.

My sight had begun to develop, and the external world was taking shape for me. At the same time, a decision gradually formed in my mind, becoming firmer and firmer, that one day I would be able to see clearly what was around me. Isaac had promised that in about six months or so I would have good eyesight. That was not quite the way it turned out, but my eyes improved enough so that I was not disappointed. One is not always aware of improvement while it is taking place, but I could tell that my eyes were getting stronger and would continue to do so. For one thing, I was reading much easier with my special magnifying lens. Not only that, I had begun to read with both eyes. My weaker left eye no longer intruded a blurred image into my field of vision as I focused on each letter. It had become strong enough to take an active role in the vision process. I think that probably the nerve centers in the brain had also begun to adjust to the new improved situation. My nystagmus condition, which was really quite bad, had lessened enough so I could control my eye movements somewhat. I was on my way to a completely different life.

I never stopped working on my eyes even while sitting in classes. Listening to the teacher, I would shift my eyes from one bell to the other in the front corners of the classroom. I was constantly moving my eyes from point to point; for by now they were strong enough to benefit from this. Often I would palm, especially during music class, where I could sit and palm for 45 minutes while listening to the lectures and symphonies.

One day my geography teacher asked me, "How do you expect to get a good grade if you're always doing eye exercises and not listening to me?" I told her I was doing both at the same time, but this only flustered her. "How can you move your eyes and still hear my voice?" She must have realized how ridiculous this question was, especially when I pointed out that people use their eyes and ears at the same time all day long. Even if they were a little disturbing to my teachers and classmates, the exercises were a necessity to me. And a few teachers and students accepted what I was doing.

I decided to take a course from a vocational massage school in order to improve my bodywork techniques. Unfortunately all I learned was that Miriam knew more about massage than the instructors. They taught us a rigid program of techniques – some were quite useful, but most were not. They never mentioned paying attention to what an individual person really needs. They didn't teach, for example, what position the therapist's body should be in while working on a patient, and they never mentioned different types of touch for different bodies or the importance of the therapist's own relaxation and presence. Though I took the course for six months, I decided not to apply for the massage certificate which was offered. The main thing I gained from this course was a sense of confidence in what I was already doing. I also enjoyed the free massages I got when we all worked on each other.

By then I was seeing several people for massage and movement sessions – people I met on the beach, people Miriam sent, and people they knew – and some of them felt strongly that they should pay me for the work. I had always refused, but after I completed that massage course I began to feel that it might be all right to accept payment.

A few weeks before graduation, Miriam called me. I was always happy to hear from her. She told me about a young man named Danny, only recently arrived in Israel from Iran, who was having difficulty walking because of progressive muscular dystrophy. She said his condition was quite severe, and she hoped I would see him.

A few weeks later Danny called me and asked if there was anything I could do for him. "My situation looks bad. All the doctors say there is nothing that can be done. Are you sure you can help me?" I told him about Eli, who, at that time, was still improving steadily. Danny was quite impressed, so we set a time to meet.

The first time I saw Danny I thought he was just a boy. I was only a year older and a little taller, but he seemed about half my size. His face wore an expression of distress, and his hands trembled, yet there was something charismatic about him. He was honest and direct, and full of intensity. During the next few years, Danny became not only my patient, but also my teacher and my closest friend.

I examined him and tested the strength of his legs. All of his toes curled upwards because the muscles weren't strong enough to hold them in place. His legs were very thin, the thighs even thinner than the calves. His stronger leg, which bore most of his weight when he stood and walked, was hard with contracted muscles. His fingers were as thin as a baby's, and his arms were almost fleshless. He could lift them only as high as his chest. His shoulders were so emaciated that if you pulled on his arms you could dislocate his shoulders. His face was thin, and there was something miserable and frightened in his expression.

Muscular dystrophy is a progressive disease that causes the muscle fibres to degenerate. Like Eli, Danny suffered from the Duchenne type of muscular dystrophy, which is always fatal. The cause of muscular dystrophy is unknown.

Danny and I discussed a strategy of treatment, and I told him, "You can definitely be cured!" He looked at me in amazement. He wasn't sure he could believe me, but even the prospect of a possible reprieve from degeneration and death seemed like salvation to him.

During our first two sessions I did all the work. I showed Danny how to rub his hands together to warm them, but at first he was only able to do this a few times before becoming exhausted. I massaged his fingers to stimulate them and increase the circulation. I worked for many hours on his arms and shoulders, gently massaging and rotating them. After several sessions, Danny's strength increased. He could rub his hands together for a few minutes, succeeding in making them warm.

Miriam had told me that a person should not remain passive during a massage because then he would be receiving stimulation but doing nothing to distribute or release the energy which massage brings. During our third session, I asked Danny to do some simple motions while I worked on him, such as moving his head from side to side or bending and straightening his knee.

Danny's abdomen was tense and hard. I taught him to breathe through his nose, and this helped expand and relax the abdominal muscles and diaphragm. But his legs needed the most work, particularly the stronger leg, whose contracted muscles were hard as a rock. It took several months before his legs could relax, but when this happened his whole body began to relax. His breathing, which had been extremely shallow, gradually deepened.

Then I tried to massage his head. At first he couldn't bear to be touched there. When he was seven years old, he'd lost the hearing in one ear following an auto accident, and shortly after that the m.d. symptoms began to appear. It amazes me that none of his doctors suspected any connection between the accident and his disease.

Whatever the cause, Danny's disease first appeared at age seven. It seemed to stop for a time while Danny was growing rapidly, but during his adolescence the deterioration process became obvious. By the time he was seventeen, when I met him, he had so much difficulty walking that he was almost ready for a wheelchair. After we came to know each other, he told me that he had decided to kill himself rather than ever use a wheelchair. He refused to lead a life as a cripple. Duchenne muscular dystrophy leads to a slow death with the patient eventually becoming too weak even to breathe.

Danny was a very special person, and a very troubled one. He told me that life is as meaningless as dust and he saw no reason to live. He was drawn to philosophers whom he found pessimistic, such as Sartre and Camus. For him life was nothing but a prison and death would be a release. After we worked together for a few months, Danny began to see some results, and his attitude improved remarkably. Suddenly, he saw that there might be a way out. He looked upon his work with me as a possible reprieve. When he was able to walk a little more easily and lift his arms twice as high, he began to believe there might be some chance of a cure.

Danny was disciplined in working on himself. After each session, and every day, he exercised for four hours. He developed his own system for working on himself. While watching TV or listening to music, he did very simple movements for as long as half an hour each. He worked on his hands, arms, shoulders, legs, stomach, and chest, and he massaged everywhere he could reach. After three months, Danny decided to stop working with me and continue by himself. For the next nine months he worked alone and refused to see me. He considered his work on his body as a kind of sculpture, and he didn't want to show it until he was satisfied with the results.

My next muscular dystrophy patient was Yankel, a gold-smith by profession. One day my grandfather dropped by my family's apartment to tell me that he had recommended me to a "one-legged man who wanted a massage," adding that it was lucky for me that the man had just one leg because that would mean half the work for me. He thought this was quite funny. I said, "If this man is one-legged, he needs more than just a massage. He will need some specialized treatment." Grandfather answered irritably, "Are you telling me how to do massage?" (He knew nothing about massage, but assumed since he was older he must know more about everything.)

"Well since you're such an expert, why don't you teach my massage class?"

"It would take fifty years for you to learn what I know," he responded. "Here is his phone number. Don't forget to use talcum powder."

Yankel called me a few days later. He told me he had progressive muscular dystrophy, and I agreed to come to his house. When I arrived, his wife told me, "There is no medical treatment that can help Yankel, but we are willing to try anything." Then Yankel entered the room with braces on both legs and supported by two canes. Though his legs were extremely thin, he was not "one-legged" as Grandfather had said.

I immediately began to work on his legs, and the massage gave him immense relief. His breathing became easier. His legs and feet, which were cold and stiff, now felt warm and relaxed. After I finished, without asking what I charged, Yankel wrote out a generous check. His appreciation of my work really bolstered my confidence.

Yankel was eager to continue the treatment. Soon I became a regular visitor at their home. They were warm Romanian people and generously welcomed me as a member of their family. I showed Yankel gentle exercises for his legs and advised him to keep them in motion as much as possible, as his job was sedentary. Since his calves were very thin, I advised him to move his feet in rotating motion to build up the calf muscles; to visualize that motion for a period of time; and then to rotate the feet again. I instructed him to make very small movements with his toes all day, to strengthen the foot and calf muscles. It was hard for him to fully bend his knees, so I told him to lie on his back and turn his feet from side to side, increasing the circulation and so building up the calf muscles, until after eight sessions he was able to bend his knees. Then I had him lie on his back, bend the knees with the feet on the floor, and make circles on the floor with his feet, moving the knees indirectly. I massaged him gently and rapidly to increase circulation. Another technique was to place my fingertips on a muscle and shake my hands so rapidly that the muscle vibrated, which created the feeling of electricity. Yankel improved rapidly, showing unmistakable gains in the strength and size of his leg muscles. His feet became more mobile and limber, and his balance while standing improved. After two months, he began to walk without the leg braces, and then he decided to give up one of the canes.

In fact, Yankel's improvement was so great that he became overconfident. One day as he was walking down the stairs, he threw one leg out to the side, the way he had to when he walked with braces on. The fragile leg slammed against the wall, and without the iron brace to protect it, it broke easily. This was partly my fault. I had appreciated his eagerness to improve – I remembered how badly I wanted to get rid of my glasses – but I didn't realize how ingrained his old walking habits were. I had shown him how to walk properly, lifting each foot and carefully placing it down, but since he still had the habit of throwing his leg out to the side, he ended up in a cast.

He wore the cast for six weeks, and I came to work on him often. He was always happy to see me. After the leg recovered, Yankel wore his braces for a while, and then gave them up again. Though he found it difficult to walk properly, he did pretty well . . . until one day, while he was exercising holding on to a chair, he started showing off for his wife how much he could do. He pretended to kick her, and he lost his balance, fell down, and broke his leg again! This time he was in a cast for three months.

In spite of these setbacks, Yankel continued to bounce back. He enjoyed doing the exercises, and they benefited him. His legs grew thicker and stronger, and one day he said to me, "You know, Meir, you owe me some money."

I became very nervous. "What did I do? What money?" I asked.

"The money I keep paying my tailor to refit my pants." Yankel had lost 30 or 40 pounds from all the exercise. The weight loss was helpful for him, as it had been difficult for him to support his heavy upper body with such skinny legs. He had gone through four size changes in four months!

I took Yankel walking on the beach a few times, and his strength and confidence increased, perhaps too rapidly. However, his enthusiasm turned out to be greater than his patience, and Yankel found it difficult to settle for gradual improvement. With two leg fractures and the prospect of only slow progress, he lost interest in working on himself. I was sad about this, for I felt Yankel could have recovered completely.

Even though I was frustrated about Eli and Yankel, I knew that each of them had taught me a lot about the nature of neuromuscular disease and about the necessity of patience and perserverance. I was eighteen and just out of high school, and already I had had three muscular dystrophy patients. Friends and relatives began to tell each other about my work, and I soon had something of a "practice." Suddenly more than twenty people were coming to me for massage, exercise, and treatments – with many varieties of muscular, spinal, and neurological problems. The more people I worked on, the more sensitive my touch became. Miriam had taught me that everyone is different and that I would have to intuitively adjust my touch and my exercises for each person, and more and more I found that I could do this.

I had come to understand that a therapist should never press on the muscles to the point of extreme pain. Especially in seriously ill patients, this can damage the nervous system and sometimes the whole body. Touch must be pleasant, not painful. Pressure may be increased gradually, as a person is ready for it and able to take it. A therapist must have very sensitive hands to know which touch is called for in each situation. I felt grateful to have studied Braille for all those years and developed the sensitivity of my fingers.

There was no magic secret. I wasn't some fantastic healer who suddenly had hands full of electricity and uncanny power. I had to work on myself constantly, and I needed to massage my hands often, particularly before working with patients. My hands, which had been weak, were growing stronger. I sensed that I was beginning to develop something new – a unique approach to the body.

Chapter 5

Vered

Because I was now working with patients, the issue of "credentials" arose. Several friends and family members told me that I could be jailed for "practicing medicine without a license." So, the summer following high school I began to look into schools of physical therapy. One admissions director told me that I couldn't study at his school because of my vision problems. Another was so outraged by the work I was already doing without a license that she said her school wouldn't consider my application.

Bella, my sister, had been living in San Francisco for a couple of years, and she thought it might be easier for me to get accepted into a school in America. I liked her idea, but it was out of the question. We simply did not have the money.

One day my Aunt Esther, Uncle Moshe's widow, telephoned. She had been completely opposed to all my work on my eyes, and then to my work with other people. But seeing my determination to continue, she offered to help me get a professsional degree in physical therapy. It wasn't that she suddenly approved of my work; she just wanted me to become someone respectable. In the past, she had suggested that I become a professor of Biblical studies or literature, but I had refused. When she finally understood that I had chosen a different direction, she decided to help me pursue it – but on her terms.

"I can't afford to send you to the United States," she told me, "but you could go some place closer, like Italy. If you can't study in Israel, then you shouldn't waste your time here." I was grateful for her offer. Since she had vigorously opposed my work for more than a year, her about-face was especially welcome, even though I knew her motivation was not a real interest in my work, but her desire to make me a "somebody." Even though I resented her motive, I felt she was right that I should take the opportunity to study abroad, and so I accepted her offer.

I prepared to leave for Italy. I studied Italian and registered with the Italian consulate. After four months of planning and a month's delay during the Yom Kippur War with Syria and Egypt, I set off for Italy. Twelve days later, I was home again.

It turned out that the school's acceptance conditions hadn't been made clear to me by the Italian Consulate. There were 270 candidates for twenty openings, eleven of which were filled before I arrived. I also learned that a degree in an Italian physical therapy school is not recognized outside of Italy.

I had left with the equivalent of $450, a generous sum at the time, and I returned with more than half of it left. My family told me privately that I'd been foolish not to take the opportunity to travel around Europe and have a vacation. But I felt that I had gone with a serious purpose, and I really didn't want to spend my aunt's money on a vacation. The abrupt change of plans was somewhat disappointing, but I was happy to be home. There was much to do.

Aunt Esther began to urge me to pursue another direction. She again took up the idea that I should become a professor of literature or philosophy. I told her that this was of no interest to me at all, and that I had my own goals and was very eager to pursue them. She insisted, "You have no direction. What you are doing is a waste of time."

I finally told her that I would rather be a masseur in a sauna than give up my work. "That's disgraceful," she shouted. "You talk like a low class bum." I was amused that my aunt, a founder of the Israeli Socialist Worker's Party, was suddenly so class conscious.

Nothing would change her mind. Even Savta agreed with her. "Esther is absolutely right. You should study literature and stop trying to make a living scratching other people's backsides." I was deeply hurt that even she felt this way, but there was nothing I wanted to do more than what I was doing.

I had grown steadily more successful in my work, and I met more and more people who were interested in it. It was easy for this to happen in Israel, because we are a very communicative – should I say nosy? – people, always interested in what others are doing. It was mostly from my family that I got arguments.

In fact, I was quite pleased with the direction of my life. I even had a real girl friend, a beautiful girl named Yaffa, who listened to my problems with sympathy and love. Her compassion helped me carry on in spite of all the stress. My work continued to be a great source of satisfaction.

Miriam always did her best to help me. The period when she was avoiding me turned out to be brief. One time she arranged for me to meet a licensed physical therapist who worked in a hospital, and he suggested that I try to get into a school of physical therapy for the blind, in England. This sounded like a good idea, but for now I wanted to stay in Israel.

In the Fall of 1973, I enrolled at Bar Ilan, a religious university outside of Tel Aviv. I wanted to get into the biology program, but all of the science departments were full by the time I registered, so I enrolled in the philosophy department.

This of course pleased my family, and I was happy enough. I had always been interested in philosophy, particularly Jewish philosophy, and there was an excellent department at Bar Ilan. My plan was to enter the biology program as soon as there was an opening.

One day at Bar Ilan a beautiful, black-haired Moroccan woman sat down beside me in the cafeteria, offered me a cookie and a cup of coffee, and quite forwardly asked, "What do you do besides study?" She told me her name was Vered, and I told her a little about my work on my eyes and my work with patients. She asked me, "Do you think you can help me? I have polio." "Of course!" I told her. We agreed to meet at my house the following day.

Vered had had five operations on her affected leg. During one operation, a piece of cement was implanted in her big toe to keep it straight. Her thigh muscles were very thin, and the calf and buttock of her weak side were almost fleshless. This forced her to walk and stand with all of her weight on the other leg. Walking was so painful she had to stop and rest every five or six steps.

She had frequent paralyzing headaches which kept her out of class. Boring lectures especially caused her great physical discomfort. She was also too shy to enter the lecture hall if she was even a few minutes late. She was a perfectionist in everything she did, and if she could not do something perfectly, she would give up for any small reason.

Vered's family was very poor and she hated this. Her father was disabled and neither of her parents worked, so the family was supported by government welfare. Vered herself earned a little money working after school.

Because of her charm and intelligence she made friends easily, but she always felt she was deceiving people. Her relationships seemed wonderful at first, but then she would gradually close herself off. There was some fear in her that made it impossible to fully open up to others. Perhaps this was because of her illness or her poverty. Whatever it was, this complex and contradictory person was the most attractive woman I had ever met. She had a mysterious kind of beauty, as you might imagine belonging to a woman of ancient times, with a smile like the Mona Lisa. She was especially pretty in a good mood, but her moods were very changeable.

Vered was also the most intelligent person I have ever met. It was not just her extraordinary range of knowledge and nearly perfect memory, but Vered had a complete honesty and openness to new things. She could always listen, and could always understand new ideas – more than just what was said, also what was behind it. She was therefore reluctant to look too closely at herself, afraid of her own clear and uncompromising insight. She could appreciate the good things in her character, but she was often dismayed by her own behaviour, and was disturbed when she could not control it. She found life to be sometimes wondrous, but mostly exhausting and impossible.

Vered had to spend whole days and nights in bed, para-lyzed by pain, depression and fatigue. Most people occasion-ally wake up tired, not wanting to face the day, but Vered felt this way most of the time. And the more she stayed in bed doing nothing, the worse she felt about herself and the world.

And yet, with all her frustrations, she kept on making new friends and welcoming new experiences. She seemed to step forward into the world with great confidence, but under-neath, her spirit, like her body, was frail and uncertain.

When Vered came to my home for the first session, I began by testing her weak leg. She could not even tolerate my lightly touching her kneecap because of the pain from the surgery. At the slightest touch, she cried out. The leg was twisted to one side because the muscles were too weak to hold it straight. All the operations had been harmful to her. It made me want to cry to see this weak and wasted leg, destroyed by the knives of surgeons. Yet I knew that she

57

could be helped tremendously and that we would have to begin by building up her weak leg. I showed her a couple of simple exercises, and we agreed to meet again.

I saw Vered several times at school before our next session. She asked whether I needed any help in reading, and when I said yes, she willingly sat and read to me from my textbooks. Her voice was clear and lovely.

I took Vered to meet Miriam, and Miriam too was charmed by her. She showed Vered a Czechoslovakian book for dancers, illustrating correct and incorrect postures of standing, sitting, and walking, and demonstrated some exercises which she thought might help Vered. One was a belly dancing technique which consisted of rotating the hips in isolation from the rest of the body. Miriam felt that Vered was someone who understood this work as few people can, and she appreciated our work together.

Vered was unbelievably sensitive to pain; even an affectionate squeeze of the hand could bring her to the point of tears. The pain in her leg was terrible. It hurt her when I worked on her, but she made a great effort to endure it. I used oil to decrease the friction, and I showed her how to breathe deeply which helped her relax a little and thereby reduce the pain.

I asked Vered to swing her arms up and down rhythmically while slowly moving her head from side to side. This released the tension in her shoulders and neck that naturally accumulates in people who have difficulty walking. Then I had her move one foot at the same time. Her foot could move only slightly, but by the end of an hour, her circulation was so much better that I was able to touch the scarred area of her knee without her feeling much pain. She told me she felt as if she were waking up from a horrible dream. After several more sessions, Vered began to notice that my touch was only occasionally painful, and then only where the deepest incisions had been made. The tissue beneath those scars was still deeply damaged, and some of the bones had never completely healed.

In our next few sessions together, I began to massage her leg under water in the bathtub. Warm water relaxes the muscles, and movement under water is easier. Some of Vered's muscles which normally could not move at all, could move in the water, where there is less gravitational resistance. After three months, she was able to bend and straighten her knees evenly in the water; and in six months she could do this out of water.

Vered did her exercises with the kind of determination I'd seen previously only in Danny and myself. She had a natural kinesthetic awareness, unlike anyone else I had ever met. After only two sessions, she was already creating new exercises to complement the ones I was giving her.

When she walked, Vered's knee had a tendency to slip backwards and "lock", holding the leg rigid. This put a lot of pressure on the knee, jarring it with every step. It was caused by the weakness of the muscles around the knee, and Vered and I concentrated on strengthening those muscles. One exercise she did for hours was to lie on her stomach and slowly raise and lower the calf of her weak leg. She then progressed to moving the calf in a rotating motion, slowly and gently working all the muscles around the knee. From being scarcely able to lift the leg at all, Vered increased the range of the movement until she could touch her buttock with her foot.

She also began to do self-massage, especially on the knee. Miriam always told me that before doing massage it is best to rub your hands together until they are warm, and that the best way to do this is with the fingers interlocked while rubbing the palms together in a rotating motion. With her hands warm, Vered would massage her knees. She did this almost constantly.

Vered especially loved the belly dancing exercise. Her pelvic muscles were painfully contracted and one hip was higher than the other, and this exercise gently loosened the pelvis and the hips. Her pelvic tightness came from the same source as most of her other problems: the imbalance in her movement caused by the weak leg. This imbalance caused some muscles to be overworked and strained and others to be neglected and atrophied. The goal of her treatment was to create equilibrium. This was quite a job, since one leg was less than half the thickness of the other, all the way up to the hip.

Although polio is a rare disease these days, looking at the problems of a polio victim can teach us about other diseases as well. Orthopedic surgeons regard polio as a mechanical problem, as if these patients were malfunctioning machines. They cut into muscles, lengthening some and shortening others, breaking bones, transferring bits of joint from one limb to another. They seem to have the sensitivity of mechanics working with cars. In polio cases, the muscles being operated on are weak and atrophied and do not have adequate nerve function or blood circulation. Surgery only decreases their ability to function even further.

Many physical therapists try to activate a polio patient's muscles, but they do not emphasize balanced movement. Patients are told to bicycle or swim or do some other "therapeutic" exercise, but nothing is done to change their habitual ways of moving and using their bodies, their breathing, or their mental conceptions about movement. Instead of suggesting fundamental changes, physical therapists often try to help their patients improve by prescribing strenuous activities. They encourage heavy use of already strong limbs, rather than trying to strengthen the weak ones, for the simple reason that they do not think that this is possible. It is similar to the way my teachers wanted me to neglect my eyes. Today we are seeing the results of this imbalanced approach in heart and stroke patients, who suffer from these ailments as a result of what doctors call post-polio syndrome. This condition seems to be caused by overexertion of one part – an arm or a leg – of a polio paitent's body during the course of therapy or exercise.

Vered and I were trying to change the entire way her body worked – to build up muscles which had partially atrophied and to encourage the use of hitherto unused muscles to do the work of those which *had* totally degenerated. We tried to balance her movement so that the two legs would work together, equally and in coordination.

Vered did this with physical exercises and with mental awareness as well. When she released some part of her body from its habitual tension, she realized that she could indeed change her condition for the better. This idea transformed her attitude towards herself and her disease. *A small shift in attitude can make the difference between improvement and deterioration.*

Vered's exceptional intelligence and ability to assimilate new ideas was an asset in her therapy. She was always creating new exercises for herself, which I was then able to use with other patients with excellent results. I would ask her to visualize that her weak leg was strong and healthy and to picture herself walking as though she had two normal legs. The results were astounding. The difference in size between the two legs became visibly less. Like almost everyone with weak legs, Vered would tense her arms and shoulders when she walked. Through breathing and slow leg exercises, alternating the two legs so neither would become tired, she released much of this tension.

We often went to the beach to exercise, first walking in shallow water to accustom her to the movement of the waves and then wading in up to her waist. There she would stand, lifting one knee at a time to hip level. Out of the water she could hardly lift her leg at all, but in the water it was easy. This trained her weaker leg to lift itself with its own muscles and helped break her habit of dragging it along when walking on land. The muscles were there; they just needed the right conditions to develop. From needing to rest every 5 or 6 steps, Vered's strength increased to where she could walk as much as three miles without discomfort. She had to work up to this distance gradually, and her muscles ached as she increased the distance. But she learned to relieve the pain and fatigue of overused muscles through gentle stretching exercises and massage. Her improvement was nothing short of phenomenal.

There came a time when I no longer needed to *search* for new exercises; they would just "come" when I needed them. I would meditate on what I was trying to accomplish while working on myself and inspiration for new exercises would come – exactly the right exercises for my back, my legs, my eyes. This also began to happen with regard to my patients. By attuning myself to them and to their needs, I knew what to do with them.

The needs of handicapped people are basically the same as those of anyone else. We must activate parts of the body which are dormant and unused and strengthen the rest of the body in order to create balanced and proper functioning. When handicapped people start to work on themselves, their movements are often abrupt, strained, and insensitive. When they massage themselves, they usually do so very roughly at first. It is especially helpful for handicapped people to learn to massage others before trying to massage themselves. After learning to be sensitive and caring towards another person's body, it is easier to extend the same consideration towards yourself. This is especially true of handicapped people, who often feel hatred towards their own bodies.

Vered introduced me to her friend Channi, who also had polio. Channi had already consulted a number of "healers" and wanted nothing more to do with them, but Vered convinced her that I was not a "healer," but a teacher of movement, so she agreed to meet with me. Like Vered, she had been stricken with polio as an infant. Her right leg was the stronger one – she called it "my beautiful leg." Her left leg was rigid and thin as a stick, and she called it "my interesting leg." The "interesting" leg had survived nine operations. Her ankle had become so weak that to prevent the foot from hanging loosely the surgeons installed a piece of her hipbone in it. This enabled her to walk without a leg brace, but she could not bend the ankle or move the foot.

Channi was attractive, but the damage to her leg had injured her self-esteem. She walked with a cane, and, as if this made it impossible for her to be pretty, she was quite careless about grooming and dress.

Like Vered, Channi's weak leg was extremely sensitive to pain. In order for her to tolerate more than a half-minute massage on that leg, I had to constantly change the kind of touch, sometimes tapping, sometimes stroking, sometimes tightly and quickly pinching, always modulating the firmness of the touch. As her tolerance for this increased, the massage brought more circulation to the injured areas, helping them feel more alive.

Channi's leg had a tendency to become hot, especially when she walked too far or sat in an awkward position. Most polio patients have legs which feel cold to the touch, due to lack of circulation. In her case, however, tension caused the blood to flow to the surface, keeping it from reaching the deeper tissues. I massaged her leg gently with a vibrating motion such as I had used on Yankel, and the accumulated fluid which had caused her leg to overheat slowly dispersed. Massage can regulate body temperature whether the body is overheated or chilled, since either one can be caused by poor circulation. Channi learned to do this for herself, and this was her first success in the therapy. Although she had been skeptical, once she began to see some improvement, she was eager to continue with the treatment. As she spent more time working on herself, I noticed that she also took better care of her appearance.

Channi and I frequently went to the beach to exercise. Even if only for the sunshine and cleansing sea air, this would have been healthy for her, but my main purpose was to help her adapt to different walking conditions. I wanted her to learn to walk in sand, where the foot sinks in at each step and you must lift your leg high to pull it out. Polio patients typically drag their legs from the hips rather than lifting them off the ground, so learning to walk on sand is very helpful. It was also helpful for Channi to learn to walk in the waves near the shore and to do leg exercises in the water, either sitting in shallow water, or standing with my assistance. It is a challenge for any polio patient to keep balanced and upright while standing in the surf.

Channi found it very difficult to walk in the sand. She lost her balance and fell with each step. It was the same in the water – a wave that would not affect a toddler would knock her over. So we approached these goals gradually, step by step. I gave her breathing exercises, massaged her legs before and after she tried to walk, and had her "walk" in the sand on her knees. I even stretched her legs by dragging her along the beach by her feet.

Little by little, her balance and strength improved. After about a dozen sessions at the beach, she could stand upright in the water and walk in the sand for ten yards without falling. As a result, she could walk much better on solid level ground with her cane, even though her foot was still completely immobile.

Channi's greatest improvement was in her thighs. I taught her to kneel with her heels under her buttocks, and then separate her legs and sit on the floor between her heels. From there she would rise up onto her knees, then lower herself again. This forced her to use both thighs equally. In ordinary movement, she had hardly moved the thigh of her weaker leg at all.

The most effective exercise by far for Channi was a mental, not a physical, one. To help her develop movement in her affected ankle, which had been completely immobile since her doctors had inserted a piece of bone in it to straighten it, I told her to rotate her stronger ankle and at the same time to visualize the other ankle rotating. When she first tried this, she told me she felt pain in the paralyzed ankle, as if it were actually moving. I told her this was a very good sign, and to continue. It took six months of faithful practice, but after that time Channi did develop a limited mobility in her ankle. It was then that she gave up her cane – forever. (When I returned to Israel, many years later, Channi came to a workshop I offered, and told me with pride that her cane has been sitting unused in the closet for more than ten years.)

I soon began working with a third young woman who also had polio. Frieda's condition was even more severe than Channi's or Vered's. Both of her legs were paralyzed, and her abdominal muscles were extremely contracted from having to work for the legs. She suffered from chronic digestive disorders, as do many polio patients, because of cramped and imbalanced abdominal muscles.

Frieda had a serious back problem. Early in her childhood her doctors had noticed that she was unable to hold her back straight, and were concerned about the possibility of progressive degeneration of the spine, so they implanted a platinum rod in her back. She had braces on both legs and on her neck. When I tested her I discovered that one foot seemed to have some potential for movement and that the knee of the same leg could also move slightly. I thought that this could develop later into enough of a motion to activate and strengthen the leg and eventually eliminate the need for a brace.

Frieda improved with my therapy to the point where she could move her foot a little, and then just as she was developing some movement in the stronger leg, she stopped coming to me. Instead she began to see a Feldenkrais therapist who concentrated on improving her back muscles so she would be more comfortable. He didn't even try to improve her legs. I have seen this again and again – someone who experiences a little improvement becomes frightened and withdraws from it.

I learned a great deal about working with the handicapped from Vered, Channi, and Frieda. Most people do not use their bodies properly and have a strong resistance to learning how. This is especially pronounced in the case of the handicapped. They try to separate themselves from the part of the body which is crippled, so it is hard for them to work on those areas.

My task was to try to help them come into touch with bodies from which they had become alienated. I was trying to help them regenerate functions which they had given up hope of ever regaining, or even to gain functions which they never had before. I was discovering something about the psychology of illness, as well as the physiology. I learned that a person must be *willing* to recover in order to overcome limitations.

Chapter 6

Our first center

My practice continued to grow. One of my patients, Lyuba, was acquainted with the director of the Vegetarian Society, the main organization of the health and nutrition movement in Israel. Lyuba told him about me, and he invited me to give a lecture there.

I was thrilled! I hadn't lectured before, and I looked forward to speaking publicly about what I'd been doing. But the prospect of my first lecture was short-lived. When I met with the society's director to make the arrangements, he discovered that I was not a vegetarian myself, so he withdrew the invitation and suggested that I meet with several of the physicians at the society's clinic instead.

This was how I met Dr Frumer. Dr Frumer had suffered two heart attacks, and realized that he had to change his ways to prevent another. He underwent a twenty-day fast, and this lowered his blood pressure and normalized his weight. After that he began exercising twenty minutes each day, eating a balanced, vegetarian diet, and leading a less stressful life. His improvement was immediate, and he became a staunch advocate of exercise and good nutrition. This was not well received by either his patients or his superiors, who preferred the usual alleviation of symptoms by drugs and surgery. A few of the patients welcomed the new methods and actually wanted to change their lifestyles, and his methods worked for them. Most of them, however, were angry and upset with the suggested changes. They either didn't want to change, or were convinced that drugs had to be the most effective treatment. They complained to the village clinic where he worked about his unorthodox methods (juice diets, fasting instead of antibiotics to reduce fever, and so on). His superiors listened to these complaints, but turned a deaf ear on his success stories – even one case of gangrene that he had successfully treated through fasting! They simply told him he could follow standard medical practice, or leave.

He resigned his practice and came to the Vegetarian Society. Here he found a niche for himself, primarily as an advocate of a well-known reducing diet especially for overweight women. His new practice was not very large, but he enjoyed the pressure-free environment where he could use simple, natural means to work with his patients. When I met Dr Frumer, he was very enthusiastic about what I had to say, and I even interested him in working on his own eyes. He eventually persuaded the Vegetarian Society to allow me to lecture and to see patients at their clinic.

At the same time, Vered and I decided to start a center where we could see patients and teach the therapy we were developing. Vered had a gift for this work, and she had begun helping me with some of my patients. We also decided to invite Danny to work with us. Although Danny was working on himself independently of me, we were still in touch. I would see him once a week for the best massage I've ever received. Muscular dystrophy patients are expected to degenerate, but Danny was actually improving. He could now not only lift his arms up normally, but he was even lifting light weights. He could climb stairs well, and his fingers had built up from being pencil-thin to being thick and strong, with incredible energy and sensitivity. I knew he would be an asset to our center!

As you can imagine, the prospect of having such a place

aroused nearly uncontrollable enthusiasm in me. Not only could we work with patients, we could work on each other, help each other with patients, and learn together; but when I talked about this with Danny, he was reluctant to join us. He didn't think he would be able to communicate well enough with his limited Hebrew, and he did not feel qualified to work with patients. I reminded him that he had the best touch of anyone, including Miriam, and told him just to look at his own body if he needed proof of his abilities. He finally agreed.

We found an apartment near Dizengoff Street, one of the main business, shopping, and entertainment areas of Tel Aviv. Vered had her own room and Danny and I shared one large room. It took me a while to earn the money to buy a sliding door to divide the room, and until we installed it, Danny and I had little privacy. Vered's room was across the corridor. None of us had ever lived away from home before, and this "Center" provided everything we wanted: rooms to work in, our own kitchen, and two large verandas, open to the sun, which Vered filled with potted flowers and plants. Vered and I worked on patients on mattresses on the floor, and I bought a massage table for Danny because it was too difficult for him to sit on the floor. The table creaked and wobbled, but it worked, and the three of us were in heaven.

The atmosphere was warm and homelike. We had planned simply to start a center for bodywork, but it soon became clear that this was also a good place for us to live. In addition to the patients who were referred to us by my family, our friends, and other patients, the Vegetarian Society clinic had signed up several patients to work with me there. Of these only two actually kept their appointments, but one of them, an older woman who talked non-stop, got many others interested in our therapy.

I liked working at the Vegetarian Society clinic. I was associated with licensed physicians who also referred patients to me. This was not only flattering, it meant I was under their protection and had the support of the 2,000–member society.

After only a few weeks there, I had a full schedule of patients. When I finally gave my first lecture, about 150 people showed up, and they were very attentive. I talked about my work with my own eyes, and about the work of Dr Bates.

The audience asked many questions afterwards. Although there were a few objections to specific things I had said, such as my blanket disapproval of sunglasses, on the whole the lecture was well-received, and I began to have even more requests for appointments.

Many of my early patients had eye problems. One of the first, Mr Vardi, had cataracts on both eyes, one of which was so mature that his lens was almost completely opaque. He could see only a little light and shadow. I doubted that his worse eye could be helped, but I gave him some exercises for his better eye. I showed him the five basic eye exercises: palming, sunning, shifting, blinking, and swinging. In swinging, you stand in one place and turn the body from side to side pivoting on the ball of the foot, and see the visual field as moving in the opposite direction. Doing this increases detail vision and makes shifting automatic.

After four months, Mr Vardi could see his fingers on his hand with his bad eye – a great improvement for him. I tried to help him further by showing him the correct way to read. Most people read a word or a sentence, or even an entire line, at a time. In order to make the best use of our eyes, we must see just one point at a time. Instead of taking in larger units such as lines or sentences, we should read word by word, letter by letter, and then point by point.

Good vision consists of seeing central details vividly and the periphery less clearly. The center point of the retina, which is called the macula, is the part of the eye which sees with the greatest acuity, but it can only see a very small portion of the visual field at a time. Therefore, in order to fully use the macula, we must constantly shift our point of focus from one small detail to the next. Eyes which see well do this automatically and unconsciously. Eyes which see poorly must consciously relearn the habit of "shifting," for they have formed the habit of staring fixedly and straining to take in the entire visual field at once, whereby the use of the macula is lost, making clear vision impossible. This is especially true in reading, where the greedy mind grabs for whole sentences at a time, straining the eyes to see in a way for which they were not designed. This can damage them permanently, even causing cataracts. Reading point by point is different from the way most people are taught, but it is the natural way the eyes work.

It was a real challenge for Mr Vardi to distinguish between letters, or even between words; he had developed over many years the habit of reading an entire line at a time. By practicing these exercises, though his cataracts did not disappear, he was able to avoid surgery, and his vision improved considerably.

An elderly woman who had had three operations for cataracts, a detached retina, and glaucoma, came to see me. She was almost totally blind; all she could see was a little sunlight. I told the secretary of the Vegetarian Society, "Sometimes people come to me too late." I will never forget his answer, "People come to you the way they are, and that's where you start." This woman did, in fact, begin to see some improvement after working on her eyes. One day, while sitting in front of the post office, she was able to see people coming and going. It was only temporary, but similar flashes of sight began to occur, and she was quite encouraged.

She brought her granddaughter, Mazel, who also had vision problems. Mazel not only learned the exercises but also took an interest in the theory behind them. She began to observe carefully how her own eyes worked and how they reacted in various situations. She felt in herself a resistance to seeing clearly, something many people with sight problems experience. Mazel realized that her extreme sensitivity to light and to such substances as chlorinated swimming pool water was caused by a general anxiety about her environment. As she learned to relax her eyes, Mazel began to take pleasure in seeing. She began psychotherapy and was able to use her eyes to become more comfortable with herself and her surroundings.

Danny, Vered, and I had different insights based on our individual experiences curing ourselves of muscular dystrophy, polio, and blindness. Together we were able to help a wide range of patients.

Danny had an acute sense of how muscles became tight and how to release them. He usually worked directly on a patient's tightest area and slowly released the tension until the tissues were softened and relaxed. Even though he only worked on a few contracted muscles, the patient's whole body would be much more relaxed. I never worked this way. A patient's tightest area was the last thing I would touch. I worked instead on all the related points. For example, for a person with a headache, I worked on the neck, shoulders, back, and stomach before even touching the head.

Danny's exercises were also much simpler and more direct than mine. Working on himself, he followed the same routine every day. He found it most important that an exercise have a direct relationship to the problem. He had to see that an exercise either built up a muscle or released it from tension. Again, my approach was different. I was most interested in the interrelationship between different parts of the body, and I tried to activate the patient's whole body, bringing him into an entirely different state of being. My movements were directed toward changing the entire rhythm of the body.

Vered leaned toward my way of working, but both she and Danny were finding techniques best suited to themselves. Just as a patient must develop his own unique approach in order to really improve, a therapist must find his own way to help each patient. The way a therapist works on a patient tells much about how he works on himself.

Danny, Vered, and I were developing a working relationship and a great feeling of camaraderie. We often exercised together and then shared our discoveries and experiences. It was as if we shared a meditation of both body and spirit. It was the deep bond of three handicapped people who had made a decision to overcome their handicaps and were working together to achieve that goal. We shared a truth which surmounted the ignorance and prejudices of the world around us. Our center was a warm, protecting place where we could be ourselves without fear of anything.

This camaraderie was not confined to us. People loved to visit our center. There were some patients who, as Vered said, stuck to our house like chewing gum. People sensed the atmosphere of security, reassurance, and optimism which arose from our conviction that we ourselves would get better. We all knew that my vision would continue to improve, that Vered's leg would grow stronger, and that Danny would completely recover.

Fortunately, when we started our center, we already had a physician's approval and support. Dr Frumer, of the Vegetarian Society, was always on our side. He referred many patients to us and he made sure that these were patients it was safe for us to work on. If he worried that a patient's condition was so serious that it might deteriorate in spite of our good work, even though we would not in his opinion have been responsible, he would not refer them, just to be sure that we had no legal difficulties.

Danny, Vered, and I realized that the natural state of the body is health. We shared this understanding with the Vegetarian Society, where the doctors also felt that the causes of illness can always be found, although they believed that diet was usually the main factor. We agreed with them that bad diet has harmful effects and good diet is beneficial, but we found that the way you move and the way you breathe are more important. We came to know that once the body was relaxed, the breathing correct, and all the joints completely flexible, it is difficult for any disease to take hold.

Often Danny or Vered, or both of them, joined me in my work at the Vegetarian Society. We had many different kinds of patients, mostly with minor problems. Many were elderly, and their problems stemmed from years of misusing their bodies. Most of them came to us not with the idea of learning to heal themselves, but simply to be "treated" or to be massaged, or even just to get a little attention. They seldom exercised at home and seemed content with the temporary relief they received during a session. As members of the Vegetarian Society, they already had some sound ideas about health, and they could appreciate our work and utilize it somewhat, even if not to its full extent.

A few were true hypochondriacs who actually did not want to be cured. They came to give our work a try, and after a couple of sessions, with their ailments safely intact, they felt satisfied that they had tried the latest treatment and it too couldn't help them.

We gave our full attention to each patient no matter how much or how little he or she appeared to respond. We always explained to each patient what we were doing and how they could help themselves. It was clear to me that no time spent on anyone was ever wasted. Our instincts and intuitions about people were sharpened. But we quickly came to recognize the kind of people for whom this work is especially rewarding. I even began to dream about founding a hospital where patients would be treated with self-healing methods and a school where practitioners in self-healing could be trained.

By this time, we already had a sizable following. My lectures and the publicity which the Vegetarian Society gave us, together with the recognition and referrals of some physicians, helped our practice grow. We began to understand and to demonstrate most of the fundamentals about illness and cures which became the basis of the self-healing method. We realized the importance of meditating on the cures of our patients. Miriam used to tell me that I needed to think for hours before each session about the person I would treat and I found this essential. Danny, Vered, and I found that our hands often knew much better than our heads what was best in a particular treatment.

Whenever a new patient came to us, first I would test her, then Danny and Vered would each test her. Usually Vered's prognosis was the most pessimistic, and Danny's the most optimistic. We never refused a patient on the grounds that she could not be helped, because Danny would always urge us to take her on. Danny felt that anyone could be cured from whatever disease she had.

One time when I took a friend with me to visit Uncle Moshe in the hospital, my friend said to me, "No matter how rich, wise, famous, or clever you are, you always end up here." This is often true, but I would now like to add: No matter how badly off you may be, or how handicapped, there is a strong power within you which can always heal you or at least make your situation better. No matter how isolated you feel, your higher self is always there to be your best friend. Knowing this, you need not feel isolated, fearful, or helpless. Our power of healing exists in every muscle of our bodies, in every brain cell, every nerve fiber, every blood vessel. We are born with the power of healing ourselves, and we only need to re-discover it. Finding this power is like opening a closet and locating what you've been looking for everywhere. It was there all the time, but you just didn't see it. We search everywhere for cures for our diseases, not realizing that there is a force within us which has an infinite capacity to heal the body. This capacity is far more powerful than any disease. Disease exists only when we overlook this healing power.

Contrary to the common understanding of disease as something bad, we discovered that disease also has a positive side.
It is an indicator of a person's state of being, and the symptoms are a clear statement about his use of his body. We
found, for example, that a patient with cataracts had probably
used his eyes rigidly for years, tensing them, staring with
them, and not blinking enough. Our job was to help him
become aware of the habits that created and were creating
the condition, and help him learn better habits. This was
necessary for a real cure to come about.

In modern life most of our activities are tightly scheduled.
We seldom have time to relax and pay attention to how we
feel and what our bodies need. Like a child, the body
demands attention and even more so when we try to ignore
it. By becoming sick or disabled, the body forces us to listen.

Most people are quite passive about disease. Modern medicine encourages us to be preoccupied with the treatment of
symptoms and to allow our bodies to be manipulated to be
like machines. It is too obvious and too frightening to look
carefully and try to discover the source of the problem. An
obvious example is the emphysema patient who continues to
smoke.

Shlomo, the old man who taught me exercises at the beach,
was someone who understood the importance of giving the
body a lot of loving attention. He worked on himself for
two hours every day. Some people who came to our center
were able to comprehend that every disease has its own cause
and its own cure: that there was a reason for their problems,
a cause for their symptoms, and a way these problems could
be resolved. These people would work with us until they
knew exactly how to work on themselves, learning what we
showed them, and learning to make their own discoveries
about their bodies and minds and what would help them.
Such people always found the best way to work on themselves. Every person suffering from a disease must discover

how to get at the cause, then how to find a cure. This process is difficult and infinitely rewarding.

Vered is a good example. I taught her to use her weaker leg instead of favoring it – to lift it up instead of dragging it along behind. It was extremely difficult for her to do this. To succeed she needed a very strong voice inside her reminding her constantly. Even after she realized that she was walking incorrectly, her resistance to change was very deep. When her walking finally showed some improvement, I instructed her to climb stairs using both legs equally. This was nearly impossible at first, since her right leg was almost paralyzed, but she learned to do it. She also learned to walk on sand, which requires bringing new muscles into play. With all of these exercises, Vered's progress was enormous. She was at the point where she could have completely overcome her limp, and at this point she hesitated. Her limp had become an integral part of her identity, and it was difficult to abandon it. I think that Vered was more aware of her true feelings than most people. None of us wants to give up accustomed ways of acting. It is difficult to be aware of these ingrained attitudes which often run counter to reason and good judgment.

Another example was a patient of ours named Reuven, who had poor blood circulation to his feet and head. When he came to us, his face was bluish, and because of impaired circulation one cheek was partly paralyzed. He also had difficulty breathing and occasional asthma attacks, as well as digestive problems, but his fundamental problem was a bad self-image.

He was only 28, but he felt defeated, having been in and out of hospitals for most of his adult life without a definite diagnosis. He had tried a number of diets and therapies. During our very first session with Reuven, his face took on a normal pinkish color from the massage and exercises we did. He began to come to us regularly and he seemed to enjoy the sessions. After only a few months, on the verge of a complete recovery – his cheek no longer paralyzed, his circulation greatly improved, his breathing free and relaxed, and the circulation to his feet quite normal – he stopped coming to our center. Sometimes at this crucial point, the patient's unconscious resistance to new patterns keeps him from making the final step to healing or success. Reuven discovered that old X-rays showed he had a hole in one lung. Even though this in no way needed to prevent his full recovery, he suddenly told us that his condition was incurable and nothing could remedy it.

At about this time, I began to observe the importance of the mind in healing the body. I had been raising and lowering my arm, very slowly, trying to relax and to breathe deeply, and I realized that I was not paying attention to the movement of the arm or to the arm's sensations. I raised it again and this time I noticed that it felt heavy and tense. I did this a few more times, and it still felt heavy. So I stopped for a while and simply visualized myself raising it. To my surprise, I found that the arm felt tense and heavy even in my imagination! I continued to visualize the movement until I could imagine the arm feeling light and the movement feeling easy. Then I tried the movement again, and the arm actually did feel a lot lighter and moved much more easily.

I was very excited about this discovery. I practiced it for a long time, visualizing the arm as light, or again as heavy, and found that I could influence my actual movement quite a lot. I immediately realized the implications that this had for my work with patients. I saw that the mind can help achieve relaxed, effortless motions, and that it is possible to bring about great changes in body functioning just through awareness.

Chapter 7

Braces for Rivka

Rivka was nine years old when she was referred to us by Miriam. She had been confined to a wheelchair since the age of two. She had been fitted with leg braces three times, but because she was unable to straighten her left knee, her walking placed so much pressure on the braces that they would always break.

Vered and I went to Rivka's home together. It was on a side street in a crowded industrial area of Tel Aviv. There was a long flight of broken-down stairs leading up to their apartment on the second floor. The small three-room dwelling housed eleven people. Rivka was the seventh of nine daughters. Her father had broken his back, disabling him permanently so that he could not work. The mother did not work outside the home either, so that the family was mainly supported by the government, although several of the sisters worked. One was a nurse, another a soldier, and the others still in school. The apartment was dark and desolate inside. Rivka was sitting in her wheelchair and looking at the floor, her eyes hidden behind thick glasses. She was a shy little girl and very small for her age.

We tested her afflicted leg. Both of her legs were very thin, and were expected to become paralyzed. Her back was stooped and had a lateral curvature in the middle of the spine. One of her arms was very weak; she could lift it chest-high only with a great deal of effort. The other arm was relatively normal. Her neck muscles were so weak that she could hardly hold her head up. Vered and I tried to convince her sisters that she could be helped. I explained that the first thing she needed was massage to improve her circulation and bring warmth to her cold limbs, and after that, some gentle movements to bring flexibility and strength. I showed them that she did have some capacity for movement, even in the semi-paralyzed leg, and that the movement in all the limbs could be improved. I emphasized, however, that improving her circulation was the first essential step. The sister who was a nurse tried to argue with me. In nursing school she had learned that circulation can only be increased via nerve stimulation, and she believed that Rivka's nervous system had been too badly damaged by the polio to provide the necessary circulation. I interrupted her, saying, "Yes, but blood flow can also increase nerve stimulation. Why don't you at least let her try our work?"

Then Vered spoke to the sisters, quietly and confidently, about the progress that she, also a polio victim, had made, first through working with me and then carrying on by herself. They agreed to try our therapy, with Vered acting as Rivka's chief therapist. Vered took the job with some reluctance. She was already working, carrying a full course load at the university, as well as working on her own legs and dealing with her own physical limitations. She was unwilling to add the long bus ride and walk twice a week to get to Rivka's apartment – this was before we had opened our Center. Vered was still not fully confident of her abilities, but with all her doubts and objections, she was excited at the prospect of a polio patient of her own, and she accepted the challenge.

Rivka's family offered Vered little support in her efforts. The full extent of their cooperation was that one of the sisters tried to encourage Rivka to do the exercises Vered showed her. The little girl was not very cooperative at first, making it clear that she enjoyed her exercises about as much as most children enjoy homework. At first, Vered found working with Rivka very frustrating, but after a time, Rivka began to show some motivation, and some changes began to take place. Her cold feet grew warm more rapidly with each treatment. She became more capable of some limited movement. She could move her feet sideways, backward and forward. Several of the muscles of her arms and legs grew stronger and appeared to be more developed. She could even lie on her back and raise her legs for several moments at a time.

Her biggest problem was her difficulty in working on herself. Rivka's home was small and crowded, offering little privacy or space in which to exercise. Vered worried that this might interfere with Rivka's growing enthusiasm. After talking it over, Vered and I decided that better surroundings were what Rivka needed most. We had just opened our Center, so we requested from Rivka's family that she come there for her treatments. At first she was able to get a ride to the Center from one of the van drivers who transported handicapped children to their special schools, and she was accompanied to the Center by one of her sisters. After the treatment we sent her home in a cab; we had cut the already nominal cost of her sessions in half, so that she could afford the cab fare. Then the van driver decided our Center was too far out of his way and refused to bring her there any more. We then had no alternative but to see Rivka for nothing, so that she could afford to take a cab both ways.

Most of the exercises we gave her at first were to be done while she was lying face down on a mat. In this position, she would raise the foot of her stronger leg, and then let it drop back onto her buttock. Then with great effort from her back and stomach muscles, she raised the leg and returned it to the mat. This exercise was very strenuous for her and she could only accomplish it after repeated efforts, alternating with visualizing the foot moving up and down. But after only a few weeks of practice, she could do this exercise for five minutes at a time before she needed to rest. She would keep this up for hours at a time, alternating exercise and rest. The muscles in her legs were so contracted that her legs were always bent at the knees. We tried to straighten them by moving them gently in rotating motion. Rivka also worked on her arms, first moving the wrist in a rotating motion, then with great effort doing the same with her elbow. It was most important for us to stimulate her sluggish circulation so that her near-paralyzed body could enjoy at least the feeling of motion.

When Rivka came to our Center, she stayed for several hours to work on herself. She sat on a couch out on the veranda, and we would often look out the window to see how she was doing. She would sit, moving her neck, then her arms, then her hands, or lie on her stomach, moving her foot in rotating motion and breathing deeply. Often we would see her simply sitting with her eyes closed, or staring up at the sky. When I asked her what she was doing, she would say, "I'm resting." I would give her five minutes to rest, and then gently insist that she get back to work. She needed many such rest breaks; nonetheless, she spent between three and four hours working on herself each time she saw us. Danny was less patient and more insistent that she work hard, and she usually worked harder when he was watching.

When we had been working with Rivka for some time, the three of us held a consultation to decide what should be the next step in her treatment. We decided that it was time for her to get braces again and begin to walk. She was suffering from a lack of stimulation, both physical and mental, and neither her home nor the special school for the handicapped which she attended could provide that stimulation. Only at our Center did she experience the freedom and activity she needed. We all agreed that it was essential that she become more mobile, that she needed to put more of herself into action. "We have to have her walking," Danny said. "If she doesn't walk, she is not going to use her muscles enough."

We talked with Rivka's family and suggested that they ask her school's orthopedist to order some braces for her. The orthopedist, however, refused to request government aid to pay for the braces. When I heard that, I decided to speak to him myself. I asked Rivka's sister Rachel, who had agreed with us that Rivka needed the braces, to accompany me and help me to persuade him.

The orthopedist seemed a bit nervous, welcoming Rachel quite formally. She introduced me as a good friend of the family. He invited us to sit down, and asked rather abruptly why we had come. When Rachel explained that we had come to repeat the family's request for braces, he became impatient. He told us that he had no intention of ordering braces for Rivka at that time, because he planned to operate on her knee within six months and she would only need a different set of braces after the operation. He refused, he said, to waste taxpayers' money on two sets of braces.

I began to explain to him that Rivka was trying a new kind of therapy, which might make such an operation unnecessary. I did not introduce myself as the therapist, but tried to describe the therapy itself. The orthopedist listened with surprising patience. He had expected nothing more than a routine discussion of requests which he would either grant or refuse. But as he listened, his interest grew and his abruptness disappeared. He was very curious about our work. I told him about some of the movements we used to relax and strengthen her muscles, and he asked with a hint of sarcasm, "So what do you need the braces for?" I explained that she needed the braces for the greater mobility they would give her, to support her process of learning to walk.

He asked me, "What are you studying?" When I answered that I was studying philosophy, he demanded, "Then why do you want to argue about medicine? It is not your field. Leave the medical matters to me."

"I'll be happy to leave medicine to you," I said, "only right now Rivka needs the braces."

He gave me a kind, patient smile and said, "Look, young fellow, you are trying to do the impossible. Her knee cannot be straightened because her muscles are in constant spasm. She has broken her braces many times in the past, because when she tries to walk on them it puts more pressure on the braces than they can withstand, even though they are designed to support a much heavier person. There is only one solution to the problem. We will surgically break her knee in order to straighten the leg. Then she'll be able to use the braces without breaking them again."

I asked him, "What if I can straighten the knee?"

"There is no way in the world you can do that," he retorted, and added, "You know, I'm smarter than you think I am," and went on to tell me quite a number of stories to demonstrate his intelligence.

"I never let anyone put anything over on me," he finished, "and I won't let you either. But I'm willing to make a deal with you. I will recommend the braces for you; then you and I will make an agreement before a notary and a couple of witnesses that if you are not able to straighten her knee within six months, you will pay for the braces."

I was not intimidated. I thanked him and said I would think about it. "Take your time," he smiled. "I'll be happy to see you again if you decide to make the agreement."

Rachel and I left his office with mixed feelings. We had made some headway, but we knew it would be very hard to predict how long it would take us to straighten Rivka's leg. It might easily be longer than six months. Just because the doctor had planned to perform his surgery at that time didn't guarantee that Rivka's leg could conform to his schedule. Straightening and strengthening her leg by our methods was bound to be a slow, painstaking process.

Most physical therapists would attempt to straighten her leg by stretching it forcefully. Rivka's muscles were too tight to be stretched in that way. I was sure that the only way to straighten it was to relax the muscles and gradually strengthen them, and that the only way to achieve that was to keep the leg muscles working and moving. I felt that the motions used in walking would be especially effective. It was absolutely necessary that she get her braces and begin to walk.

I told Rachel that even if we did not succeed in straightening Rivka's leg in half a year, at least Rivka would get her braces. I was perfectly willing to take upon myself the responsibility of paying for them if we failed. Rachel was deeply touched. Her sister Mazel, however, was not at all pleased, insisting that the government should pay for the braces. As a nurse, she was accustomed to having the government supply everything a patient needed.

With or without of the support of the orthopedist, we – Rivka, her sisters, and I – were all convinced that the braces were essential. She needed movement, variety, a new environment, an escape from the stifling atmosphere of her home and school. It was very difficult and inconvenient to always be carried or pushed in a wheelchair. She had to have braces to achieve any degree of freedom. I discussed the problem with my friends. One friend suggested that I ask the orthopedist for more time. I agreed with this, both because I doubted that six months would be enough time, and because I was afraid that the deadline might cause me to work too intensively with her, which would be hard on both of us. So I decided to ask the doctor to change his terms.

After two weeks, Rachel and I returned to the orthopedist's office. He welcomed me with a challenging grin and said, "So, what have you decided? Do we have a bet?"

I answered him, "Yes, only I want you to give me two years." His jaw dropped in amazement, followed by outrage. He told me, "Get out of here, you charlatan."

Then Rachel grew angry, and shouted at the orthopedist, "I don't want my sister to have that operation at all if you aren't going to help us now!"

85

He answered her patiently, "I'm only trying to help Rivka; all I want is what's best for her." He turned back to me. "What about eight months?" he offered.

"Forget it," I said. "We're not in a marketplace. If you give me two years she is going to have a straight leg. I'm perfectly willing to bet, though, that in eight months she'll have a noticeably straighter leg."

"No," he replied. "I'm not going to make deals with a quack. I want a straight leg within six to eight months, and if not, you have to pay for the braces." We left then, as it was clear that another solution had to be found.

Meanwhile I was in a state of shock. No one had ever called me a quack before, and I had been working on people for years. When Aunt Esther heard the story, she smiled and said, "Well, now you've learned your lesson. You'd better be prepared to hear the same thing from other people."

Rivka's doctor had refused even to consider that our work might have some validity. I felt that this was an insult, not only to me, but to the truth. Many other doctors I have met would have done everything in their power to seek out any method that could possibly have helped their patients. Even if he did not have the imagination to understand the work in theory, the results would have spoken for themselves. I hadn't really expected him to go along with my plan, but I was nonetheless disappointed and rather depressed and remained to some degree in a state of shock for a long time after this interview.

When I told Dr Frumer what the orthopedist had said to me, he was amazed and made it clear that he disagreed. It was a relief to me to know that I had the support of an established physician who understood and approved of what I was doing. I was very unwilling to repeat the experience I'd had with Rivka's doctor. But as the shock wore off, I regained my equilibrium. I was not afraid that the orthopedist would take legal action against me, even though he considered me a fraud. I realized that while he doubted my abilities and rejected my proposal, he did not actually oppose me. He simply could not support me.

That was when I realized that there is a big difference between "opposing" and "not accepting." When you cannot accept something, a part of you is aware, either consciously or subconsciously, that you are coming up against your own limitations. In the doctor's case, there was an element of fear involved. He was afraid to discover that something so completely contrary to his training, education and beliefs, might work – might be, indeed, exactly what his patients needed. He did not want to have to challenge his training and his past practice.

Even if he had wanted to actually oppose me, he would have no grounds to do so. I could show results proving the truth of my ideas. But the doctor was unwilling to even investigate my work. If he had come to watch us work on her, with gentle massage, circular movements of the joints, and slow, gradual stretching of her muscles, it might very well have changed his attitude.

We knew that we had to get the braces for Rivka in one way or another. The question was, how? And the solution came to us quite by surprise. Vered's friend Channi was living at the time with two other women, one of whom, Tirza, was the assistant producer of a weekly radio program. In this capacity, she was very interested in the work we were doing. When Tirza offered to interview us on the radio, it occurred to me that this might be an excellent way to solicit donations for Rivka's braces. I wanted to let the public know how important it was for us to help Rivka and others like her.

The time scheduled for the interview was ideal. We were to have fifty minutes on Friday evening, just after people returned home from work, and just before television programming for the evening began. It was well-publicized in the newspapers and we had reason to believe that close to half a million people would hear it. The recording of the broadcast took between five and six hours, but when it was edited down to fifty minutes, it was quite different from what we had expected. The interviewers tried to sensationalize our work. They tried to create a sort of official documentary, instead of the informal and personal interview we had actually given them.

Nonetheless, the program did make a good enough impression to attract the attention of many people. We raised more than enough money to buy the braces for Rivka, and a good part of this came from Tirza herself. After that, Rivka's development speeded up greatly.

To walk with braces, Rivka also needed to use crutches, which required that she strengthen her arms. She had been practicing imagining her hands lifting up into the air by themselves, with no effort, and this imagery began to take effect. She had once suffered from a total lack of function in the deltoid muscles of her upper arms. Now these muscles were becoming noticeably thicker and stronger, until at last she could raise her arms. When she was able to do this and had practiced it for two months, we gave her some "weights" to lift, first a grapefruit and then a cantaloupe. By this time Rivka could work on herself steadily for hours at a time, without needing constant prodding from us. Left alone, she would continue to exercise, and when we came back she would still be at it.

When she got her braces, we started to take her for walks before dinner, and then invite her to eat with us. At first she could only take about fifteen steps at a time, and I had to carry her down the few steps leading from our apartment to the street. But before long she could go down the steps by herself, and after a while she was able to walk a whole block – several hundred yards – on her own. I used to tell her not to eat French fries, which she loved, especially not from a deli near our house, where the same oil was used for several batches. But one day when she had walked the half mile to that deli, where she almost collapsed from the effort, I gave in and bought her a big bag of French fries. She ate them with a pleasure that showed she knew she deserved a treat.

In the beginning, she always needed me to be near her when she walked, to help her keep her balance and prevent her from falling. She also needed to feel my reassurance and emotional support. Later, she was able to walk alone around the block. Her walk was very slow and laborious, but inside, she was soaring. Rivka began to awaken as a person. She had been completely indifferent to herself, feeling useless and unwanted. Now, she began to feel that she was a person who really mattered. She had been almost completely immobile, able to take only a few steps with braces, or on her knees. Now she could get out into the world on her own two feet.

It was almost exactly six months after my argument with her orthopedist, about three months after receiving her braces, when her walking made a dramatic leap in improvement. She could walk half a mile in 20 minutes, where before it had taken her an hour and a half. Her walking had strengthened her knee muscles and reactivated her lower back muscles, which had been so numb and contracted that they felt like dead flesh. It became easier for us to rotate and stretch her legs, and as a result, Rivka's knees straightened until at last they had become completely straight. Rivka began to wear her braces for four or five hours a day, while before she had never been able to tolerate them for more than half an hour.

On top of that, her formerly paralyzed arms were now fully mobile and growing stronger. We gradually increased the amount of weight she could lift, until it was up to twenty pounds. After six months of wearing her braces, she could walk a whole mile. Once she had accomplished this, she worked to increase her speed until she could walk a mile in little more than half an hour – very close to the normal speed of walking.

One of Rivka's greatest triumphs was also one of mine. She came late to one of her sessions one day, accompanied by one of her sisters, who announced, "We're late because we took the bus today." Giving Rivka a look of admiration and pride, she added, "You know, this is the first time Rivka ever took the bus. She climbed the stairs all by herself." I held my tears from running down my face, but my eyes were wet. I carried Rivka up the stairs, so she should make no more effort, took off her braces, and massaged her feet and legs, which were tight with exertion. I was exhilarated at the thought of Rivka's new independence. She was like a timid little caged bird which had finally been set free.

I thought about the orthopedist's plan to break her leg. He had never for a minute believed that she could regain function in her legs, never hoped that she would develop her wasted muscles, never imagined that she could do more than take a couple of steps with her braces. Seeing Rivka come to life was a feeling that made the whole world come alive for me and for all of us. Vered said to me, "You should have made that bet after all. You would have won."

But with or without the wager, it was clear that everybody had won, not only Rivka, not only the three of us, but the world itself had won something in that there was one less crippled child. For it is my deep belief that the suffering of each afflicted person affects the whole world, and that the state of the whole world is reflected in the life of each individual.

Part II

Self-healing therapy

Chapter 8

Back problems

Over the past fifteen years I have seen more than 1,000 people with back problems of many kinds, and most have shown remarkable improvement after learning correct movement. In my experience, all back problems can be greatly alleviated or completely cured by understanding how the condition developed and, using proper exercises, breathing, and massage, relearning how to use the spine correctly.

Most doctors and health care practitioners believe that back problems are caused by misshapen spines. I am convinced that the inverse is true. Using your back and your body incorrectly is what causes the spine to become misshapen. Most people use the whole back for every motion, as if the back is a single, inflexible entity. The back is comprised of individual vertebrae and small, separate muscle groups. It is natural and healthy to use the back flexibly, not rigidly. If you use the muscles of the back to do the work of the limbs and other parts of the body, you create unnecessary tension in the back and unnecessary rigidity in the limbs. The brain gets the message that the back needs to work when it actually doesn't, and that the limbs do not need to work when they actually do.

When I first examine a spine patient, I look at how the patient walks, particularly whether the walk is balanced. Proper gait and balance require proper use of the body's exact physical center, which is located in the area around the navel. According to the law of gravity, two masses are attracted to one another by their centers. People are connected to the earth's center by their own centers. If a person always operates from his gravitational center, then the person's posture and spine will be straight and the movements of his body will be perfectly balanced. Problems such as imbalance, gait difficulties, and chronic back tension arise when the "center" of movement is shifted from the abdomen to some other part of the body.

To understand this concept, imagine throwing a softball. The force needed for this action comes primarily from the shoulder. The energy, or impetus, for throwing gathers in the shoulder and is expelled all along the arm, into the hand and into the ball, and it is this force which moves the ball. This is how the center works. It is the focal point where the energy needed for an action gathers, and the point from which that energy is directed to the rest of the body. Naturally, using our actual physical center as the "center" of movement is the easiest, least stressful, and most "economical" way to move. However, in many people, the "center" of movement has been shifted – due to incorrect movement patterns – to some other part of the body, such as the chest, neck, or shoulders. When this happens, movement will become difficult, awkward and constrained, rather than easy and natural. The energy needed for movement will be drawn from an area which was never designed to meet that kind of demand, and the false "center" will take the strain whenever a movement is done.

For many people, the center of movement is in the back of the head. The muscles and nerves in the back of the head are called upon to direct and provide the impetus and energy for movement for the entire body. This will cause the head to be drawn forward or backward from its normal upright position, tightening the neck and the spine and preventing full respiration. Chronic tension in the lower back will result, drawing the back into a distorted "S"-curve. The "S"-curve has become so common that it is considered normal, but it is in fact the source of most spine ailments. It leads to blockage of circulation and innervation to pinched nerves and tense muscles. Spinal curvature of this kind pushes the pelvis forward, cramping the abdominal cavity and interfering with the activity of the internal organs. It limits the expansion of the lungs, inhibiting full respiration. Miriam taught me to recognize where a person's "center" was by observing how they stood. If we don't stand and walk so that all our weight is distributed evenly on every part of the feet, we are automatically "off-center", and the imbalance will be reflected in all our movements. Many people walk predominantly on their heels, or on the balls of their feet, or on their toes. The part of the foot which receives the most pressure determines where the person's center is. If I walk predominantly on my toes, my center will be in my neck or in the back of my head. If I throw my weight on to the balls of my feet, my center will be in my chest, causing the upper back to curve out sharply. In some cases this may lead to a hump or sway-back. The first step in correcting such problems is mental awareness. I would explain to the person which part of the body was being used as the center, show where the actual center is, and then instruct the person to develop a kinesthetic awareness of the true center. I had them try to visualize the center and to feel its location. Sometimes simply placing the hands over the abdomen and breathing deeply would be enough. I would have them try to be aware of the feelings of constriction and strain which accompany a misplaced center of gravity, and to replace those feelings with a sense of expansion and lightness. I would ask the person to relax the head, the neck, the chest, and especially to relax whichever part of the body has been operating as the "center."

The second thing I notice is how the patient sits. Spine patients tend to sit with their backs and heads bent forward or curved backward and with their weight more on one buttock than the other. Third, I notice how the patient lies on a firm surface, whether his back is relaxed or the small of the back is tensed so that the lower back curves upwards. From these observations, I can tell how a person's back problems developed.

When I examine a new spine patient, I try to locate all the sore spots on his body and massage them until they are no longer painful. Sore spots indicate muscle tension caused by lack of movement. These are likely to be places where emotional tension is stored. Often I will find places which are extremely tight and sore which the patient did not know about until they are touched. It is important to show the patient how to breathe freely and deeply into the abdomen so that the back can expand and be in constant movement while breathing. With constant movement in the back, there is little chance the back will become tense and stiff.

My first back patient was a French Israeli named Gabi, whom I met through Shlomo at the beach. Gabi was an intellectual and a philosopher with an extremely pessimistic outlook; and he was also a compulsive womanizer. He had been married and divorced six times.

He was rarely satisfied with anything, and this expressed itself in his posture. He dragged his feet when he walked, walking with the weight on his toes, and gave the impression that his body was a burden. His center was in the back of his neck, as his back was continually hunched over, and he was often tired.

We met on and off for two years. Each time I worked on him, the massage would relax him so he felt better for a day or two, but would soon revert to his habitual, heavy way of walking. The brain would issue its familiar instructions, and the wrong muscles, those in his lower back, would become unnecessarily involved in his walking. This would cause renewed back pain, and he would begin the cycle again.

Gabi was set in his ways and did not want to change.

Like many people who are not aware of the cause of their difficulties, he continued to use a few overburdened muscles in a forced, strained way, while remaining unaware of the burden his body was to him. Massage relaxed him and helped him breathe better, but he never exercised on his own to reinforce this. Gabi was someone I wish I could have helped more, but he never really wanted to improve.

A man named David came to see us after attending a lecture I gave on vision. He believed in preventive medicine and was angry at doctors because their drugs and surgery hadn't helped his back problems at all.

David lived in a small port town near Tel Aviv and worked for the phone company. A tall man, his rounded shoulders and slumped posture betrayed how weak and small he felt. His spine had a pronounced S-curve, and his legs and stomach were very tense. His main weakness was in the middle of his back between the lumbar and thoracic vertebrae. This is often a weak area in people who suffer from low self-esteem. David was inspired by my lecture because he saw in me the triumph of someone who could have remained helpless and weak but had not. He felt he too could overcome his disability.

We taught David a series of non-strenuous movements to relax and gently activate each joint and muscle of his back. We taught him how to sit and stand properly. The best exercise was a visualization exercise which he would do after preliminary massage and exercising. He would lie on his back with his eyes closed and imagine that his head was very heavy – in fact, attached to the table – that his legs were also very heavy, and that his spine was lying perfectly flat against the table pulled down by its own weight. After experiencing this heaviness for a while, David would then imagine himself as weightless. This gave him the sensation he could float away. He would then lie on his side while I massaged his shoulders, and I asked him to imagine that I was massaging each of his vertebrae. He could feel the muscles in his back loosening and relaxing as he visualized this. Sometimes imagination is more effective than even massage for relaxing tight muscles. I touched every part of his body – forehead, skull, back of the head, cheeks, neck, and so on. I left my hands on each part for half a minute, telling him, "Be aware of this part of you. How does that feel? Be in touch with it – what sensations is it experiencing?" This helped him to get back in touch with the body from which he had become detached.

Then I asked David to be aware of all the emotional pain which was stored in the muscles of his chest and to feel the tension he carried in his diaphragm, under his shoulder blades, in his solar plexus, rib cage, and lower abdomen, and to picture the abdomen first as red and then white, as though redness were pouring into it and then flowing out again. I asked him to notice the relationship between his fingers and toes and to think about how the body connects them. He would then imagine blood rushing into his legs, all the way to his toes, then up his legs again into his stomach, rib cage, shoulders, and arms.

After doing that exercise, David always felt as if a heavy burden had been lifted. By becoming more aware of his tension, he learned how he might also relax. He encountered all the obstacles in his life and could now direct the energy which was released towards a healthier life, He became astute at noticing tension as it arose and served as his own therapist in relieving it. After only six months, David gained enough confidence and experience that he didn't need to see us anymore.

I met General Shadmi on a summer day, during my afternoon break. Most people in Israel take a break from work during the hours between two and four, when the heat becomes almost intolerable for some. Danny had just finished making lunch for the three of us. Our lunches always began with a huge slice from the watermelon I would buy daily from a man who sold them from a horse-drawn wagon. On those hot days I could have eaten whole watermelons by myself.

But just as I was about to get up for lunch, someone came through the door. He was a tall, grey-haired older man, who greeted me politely, saying, "Hello, I'm Mr Shadmi, are you Meir Schneider? I've just been talking with Noam, the Alexander teacher. We were discussing some eye surgery I'm supposed to have and he suggested that I talk to you before going through with it." "What eye surgery are you supposed to have?" I asked him. "It's an operation to correct my left eye. Do you see how it turns inward?" I came closer and looked at his eye; it did turn sharply inward, as though it were trying to look at his nose. He could not turn it to look at my finger. Then I shone a lamp into his eyes and studied them, noticing red spots on the whites, which indicated that the eyes were under a great deal of strain. "Do you have some problem with your sixth cranial nerve?" I asked. "That's right," he replied. "Well, I think we could help this without surgery," I told him. "That would be wonderful," Mr Shadmi said. "I'd do anything to avoid another operation."

During our first sessions I taught him palming, sunning, shifting, and blinking, the most basic eye exercises. I asked him to tell me about himself, and about what had caused his eye problem. He said, "It happened when I was in the Army. I was patrolling in a helicopter in the Golan Heights, during the Yom Kippur war. I was attacked and shot down, and my body was nearly torn in half. The shock of the fall was what damaged my sixth cranial nerve. After I was shot down I took my submachine gun and shot at the Arabs, and the result was seven broken ribs. The doctors only gave me a 40% chance of survival, but I recovered. I had intensive physical therapy, and then someone suggested I see an Alexander teacher. The Alexander work was really what saved my life. Every night after work I lie down on the sofa with my knees up, rest my head on a hard pillow, close my eyes, and meditate on extending my back – especially the lower back – and relaxing my muscles. And when I relax I can just feel my vertebrae settling into place. I feel like I couldn't go on without that."

It was obvious that though he had come to me specifically for eye exercises, Mr Shadmi needed body work just as urgently. He was so stiff that he even found palming difficult, because he could not lean forward while sitting. Any forward motion of his back was very difficult for him.

The helicopter accident which had severed his cranial nerve had also shattered his pelvis. Excellent surgery had repaired the pelvis to a great extent, but had left his back almost immobile. Two vertebrae had fused in the lower back. When he wanted to tie his shoes he had to lift his feet up to where he could easily reach them with his hands, because he could not bend forward. He was often in severe pain.

I massaged his back until it relaxed somewhat, then asked him to lie on his stomach and bend one knee and move the calf in a rotating motion. He tried to do this but was unable to do it smoothly; the leg moved spasmodically in little jerking motions. So I asked him instead to visualize doing the motion, and even in his imagination the leg jerked and twitched. After visualizing, he tried the motion again and found that he could do it better than before. He then repeated the visualization and found that he was able to visualize doing the motion much more smoothly. Visualization exercises show how much a person's physical and mental states reflect one another.

After this, Mr Shadmi found that his leg, and to a lesser degree his whole body, felt lighter. He was also more flexible, being able to bend the leg further back so that the calf was closer to the thigh, showing that the lower back had relaxed somewhat. By the end of our third session, Mr Shadmi's flexibility had increased so much that he was able to bend over and tie his shoes. Grinning, he said, "Well, it's back to normal life for me. I can actually tie my own shoes. It's a miracle." The exercises which had accomplished this were exercises designed to loosen his pelvis, most of which were done lying on his back. He would bend one knee and cross it over his body to touch the floor on the opposite side, and then bend it and extend it out to its own side. He would pull one or both knees up to his chest and move them in rotating motion with his hands. These exercises greatly reduced the tension in his lower back.

His work with the Alexander teacher had taught him how to relax, to release his muscles and improve his posture, and made his work with me much more effective. The Alexander method was one of the first acknowledged bodywork methods created in the West. F.M. Alexander was an Australian actor and singer who had lost his ability to perform due to a chronically hoarse voice and stooped back. While trying to overcome these problems, he looked in the mirror one day and realized that he had no kinesthetic sense of his posture – his back felt straight to him when it was actually stooped, and vice versa. The result was that he devised a method of giving mental instruction to his muscles, telling them to become long and soft, improving his posture by directing his neck to lengthen and his spine to flatten. All methods of bodywork aim to do the same in one way or another, to relax muscles, increase flexibility and awareness of where tension and blockages occur. Many also echo Alexander's assertion that tension in the therapist may be transferred to the patient.

Although Mr Shadmi did well with breathing and the stretching exercises, he was very lax about doing his eye exercises, and unwilling to make other changes I had suggested, such as changing his diet. I finally decided that I would stop teaching him eye exercises, as it was useless without his cooperation. However, I did continue to advise against the eye surgery, which could not completely correct his problem anyway, and would make it more difficult for him if at a later time he should decide to work seriously on his eyes.

It was very difficult for this busy man to find the hours he needed to work on his eyes intensively. Like most people, he was more willing to give his time to his job or to other people than to himself. But all things considered, his improvement was remarkable. Within eight sessions, he was able to bend over and touch the floor. This was mostly the result of massage. One day he came to me after he had been sitting outdoors on a bench for hours listening to a concert. He felt as stiff as the first day he had come to see me, and he thought that it would take quite a few sessions to repair the damage. But after only five minutes of intensive massage, he was able to stand up, bend over and touch his toes, with no effort or pain.

Mr Shadmi told me that he planned to continue exercising for the rest of his life. He very much appreciated his new flexibility, his deepened breathing, his increased energy and capacity for deep relaxation. I hope that someday he will take it all the way, work to improve his eyes as well as his back, and learn not to begrudge himself the hours he needs to work on his body.

Mr Shadmi is typical of modern people. We work ourselves literally to death. In the military Shadmi had worked 18 hours a day; as head of an electrical company he now worked 13. He would not take time off from work to devote to his health, much less for enjoyment. The pressure was always on.

The irony is that if a person will take the time to work on himself, the tensions of pressures of life and work become much easier to deal with. They do not go away, but the person brings much more to his activities if he is relaxed and feeling strong and capable. Usually he can accomplish more, and more successfully. However, it is difficult to impress this upon people like Shadmi, who give their lives for their work, their family and friends, their country, but cannot find an hour a day for themselves.

It is this mentality which has separated us as individuals

from the deep inner source of life. This is a great paradox; we sacrifice our lives in order to sustain them. We become enslaved by our ceaseless round of activities. Is this really living? We need to take the time to find and develop our inner resources, and then bring these resources to our work and our interaction with other people. Everything we do should be a part of our development and a step on our journey of self-discovery. Then nothing is done mechanically, but with new meaning.

I think the body is the best place to start, for the body is a central part of each person's identity. If the body is regarded with reverence and care, this attitude can be extended to the whole self. We need to learn that we are more important than our work, and caring for our bodies can train us in this attitude. Nothing should be allowed to tense our muscles or distort our spines, restrict our breathing or abuse our eyes. And we should learn to value ourselves at a very early age, for it is difficult for an adult to change the habits of a lifetime.

Isn't the quality of life as important as life itself?

One day I received a phone call from a man named Yosef who told me that his wife, Naomi, had just tried to lift both of their twins and her spine had locked, so she couldn't move. Yosef came to our center to pick me up and we drove twenty miles to their home. When we arrived, I saw stark fear in Naomi's face. Fear and pain were inseparable in her. She told me simply, "I cannot move." She was completely convinced of this. Yet I learned that she was able to get to and from the bathroom by herself. It caused her pain, but because it was a necessity, she managed to do it. But the thought of changing her position from lying on her back to lying on her side, which I asked her to do, seemed impossible to her.

Naomi felt a great relief that someone was there to help her. I began to massage her foot, and after it relaxed a little, I massaged her leg, and her abdomen, touching her gently and carefully. Her breathing was almost imperceptible at first, but it deepened as I worked. I then massaged her other leg from the foot to the abdomen, and although the pain was still there, she had almost forgotten that she couldn't move. She was able to lie on her side as I worked on her pelvis and hips. After an hour, she was able to lie on her stomach so I could work on her back.

Her lower back was so tight the contracted muscles felt like stone. In the lumbar region three vertebrae seemed almost fused. I was easily able to feel the structural effects of her muscular tension. After three hours, Naomi felt looser, and her breathing deepened naturally. By the end of our three-hour session, she sat up, although with great difficulty. She had some release from her constant pain, but I knew it would not take much for Naomi to be in pain again.

It was evening when Naomi's husband drove me home. I was exhausted from the session and went right to bed. But my sweet and soothing sleep was soon interrupted by another call from Yosef. It was 2:00 a.m. He was apologetic, but he told me that Naomi was in severe pain and asked if I could come see her again. I agreed, but immediately fell back to sleep. An hour later I was awakened by his knock at my door. Yosef was quite nervous, smoking constantly and driving very fast. When we reached their home I went in to see Naomi, who was on her back again, her face rigid with fear.

I asked her to concentrate on her scalp. I wanted Naomi to relax through a slow process of visualization. I asked her to think about the roots of her hair and the skin that surrounded them, and to allow the skin to relax. Then I asked her to imagine her breath filling her skull and to imagine the skull filling with nourishing oxygen. Naomi became aware that she was tensing her scalp, and she began to release it. While she concentrated on her breathing, it deepened dramatically.

I slowly massaged her toes to relax her foot a little. After twenty minutes of massage, I could touch her foot firmly.

Naomi was breathing so deeply that she could feel her lower back expand with each breath. The tension in her foot was connected to the tension around the compressed vertebrae. I could feel in Naomi's foot the pain she felt throughout her body. She gradually became aware of the source of it – the tension in the muscles of her lower spine. As Naomi breathed deeply, her muscles deeply relaxed, and when this happened, the pain lessened. Her pain was emotional as well as physical. Feelings of helplessness, incapability, loneliness, and inability to communicate are common to spine-injured patients.

I was now able to move her legs sideways, apart, and upwards, without hurting her. Moving her legs increased the circulation to the lower back, which was still so tense I could not touch it. When I asked Naomi to focus awareness on that area, the pain was unbearable, so I asked her to visualize her hands and feet instead and to experience their sensations. Focusing awareness in this way tends to relax the area and increase circulation both to that area and to the whole body. I massaged her calves while she lay on her back, releasing many small points of tension in the muscles. I worked on her knees, one at a time, her thighs, and then her abdomen.

It was five o'clock in the morning when I started to work on her abdomen. A little while later, I looked out the window and saw the first red light of morning starting to appear on the horizon. I told Naomi, "It's dawn already. The sun is just beginning to come up. I wish I could go outside and get a breath of air." She smiled a little. She was feeling some relief from her pain by then, and she said, "Oh, I wish I could too," and sighed. She could not see out the window, which was on the wall behind her bed. Later I said, "The dawn is getting brighter, and some light clouds are moving across the sky." Her breathing deepened as she listened to my description, and she relaxed and was able to roll over on her side. The first faint red light, which had scarcely been able to penetrate the gray of dawn, steadily brightened until it overcame the darkness and illuminated the whole morning sky. Seeing it through my eyes, Naomi became a part of it. The beautiful sunrise renewed us both. Naomi breathed more and more deeply, and her pain diminished. The sky was almost light when her pain finally left her completely. "The moment of dawn is holy," Naomi said to me.

Fearfully, but without pain, Naomi sat up, then finding that it did not hurt her, she slowly rose from bed and took three steps without tensing any of her muscles. On the fourth step her back contracted suddenly, and she nearly fell, but I caught her. I showed her how my back muscles would tense if I forced them to participate in the motion of walking and how they remained loose and relaxed if I did not. She felt how the different ways of walking influenced the muscles of my back, and immediately grasped that the same process occurred in her own back. After that, she walked without using or tensing her back muscles. Naomi walked around the bed and stood with me at the window. "It's the most beautiful sunrise I have ever seen, Meir," she said softly. All my hours of work had been worthwhile.

I continued to see Naomi regularly for a year, and at the end of that time she was completely well. Her willingness to see the cause of her problem and to learn a new way of being made this possible.

Chapter 9

Arthritis

Arthritis is a disease in which the joints – the spaces in which the bones connect to each other – become stiff and painful to move due to deterioration of cartilage, the connective tissue within the joints. Most joints are composed of hyaline cartilage, a glossy-surfaced tissue which is elastic and yet nearly as hard as bone, and fibrous cartilage, a tough elastic structure in which hyaline tissue is combined with fibrous tissue. Hyaline cartilage coats the ends of bones, allowing them to glide easily and smoothly within the joints, while fibrous cartilage cushions the impact of movement. Arthritis causes cartilage to deteriorate and eventually to disappear. In arthritic joints the hyaline cartilage loses its smoothness, becoming rough and pitted so that the bones lose their ability to glide and eventually erode at their edges.

Arthritis begins with pain, swelling, inflammation and fluid build-up in the joints, which I believe is created by the stress of damaging, incorrect movement of the joints, and also – especially in the case of rheumatoid arthritis – by a breakdown in the functioning of the immune system. Both incorrect movement and damage to the immune system may be brought on by physical and emotional stress.

Therefore our work with arthritis emphasizes re-educating a person in how to move without stress or undue impact. Through the use of relaxing exercises, we can allow the joints to move to the best of their ability, thereby reducing inflammation and draining off the fluid build-up which causes so much of the pain of arthritis in the early stages. These exercises promote the functioning of the body's innate healing mechanisms which provide for the repair of cartilage as for all other body tissues.

A sensitive touch is particularly important in treating arthritis. A variety of massage techniques and very gentle movements stimulate the blood flow, and help disperse accumulated fluids. This reduces the swelling and softens the cartilage. The therapist needs to sense exactly how much movement the joints will allow. These gentle movements should be repeated many times with great care, patience, attention, and deep breathing, to promote blood circulation into the joints. These are the keys to curing arthritis.

During my last year in Israel, Dr Raison of the Vegetarian Society sent an arthritis patient named Rachel to see me. She arrived leaning on a cane and assisted by her husband. Rachel was in her forties and appeared miserable and pain-wracked. When she saw me, she said, "You are quite young. But since Dr Raison recommended you, I suppose it is all right." We joked about this, and she seemed ready to try my treatment.

Rachel had been stricken with arthritis two years previously, and for a year it affected her whole body. Then the arthritis concentrated itself in one knee, which was swollen to more than twice the size of the other. Most osteoarthritic patients have swollen knees, but Rachel's knee was the worst I have ever encountered.

One of Rachel's doctors had recommended she have the fluid drained from her knee, but Dr Raison vehemently opposed this. She became totally distraught, and begged him to hospitalize her so she could get the fluid drained. But Raison was adamant. "It would be the worst thing you could do. You could get an infection, or even blood poisoning."

"Then give me tranquilizers, please," she pleaded with

him. "The pain is so bad I can't get even one hour's sleep at night."

"No, you must not take tranquilizers. There is one thing I can recommend you try," and he suggested our therapy, along with a severe diet of organic fruit for breakfast and only sesame seeds, tahini (sesame butter), lettuce, and cucumber the rest of the day. "This diet is unbearable," she confided to me. "The tahini tastes like mud and the sesame seeds are bitter. Those vegetables are so boring day after day." I was reluctant to criticize a diet suggested by Dr Raison, but the anxiety it produced in Rachel seemed counter-productive.

I began by massaging Rachel's back. I didn't even touch her knee. And I began showing her how to breathe deeply, and told her to visualize a color she liked. After 45 minutes of deep breathing, visualization, and massage, she was more relaxed and her knee a bit more mobile. That night she slept for three hours. Then, for several months, Danny took over her treatment. He had the gentlest touch of the three of us. With Danny gently squeezing and tapping the swollen area, Rachel's circulation began to improve and the pain and swelling in the knee lessened. She had been unable to sleep more than one or two hours per night, and she was now able to sleep six or seven hours. Rachel told Danny, "I am beginning to feel human again."

After she had been in therapy with Danny for four months, I began to treat her again. Breathing exercises were extremely helpful for her. She would visualize the air going into her joints as she breathed. In just two more months, Rachel didn't need any more treatments. I gave her many exercises to continue working on herself, including foot rotations, knee movements, and self-massage. Within just six months, her arthritis was imperceptible.

My work with arthritis patients has shown me that arthritis can be improved dramatically just by slowly and carefully moving the joints every day for several hours. If this is done faithfully, the process need not require more than a year or two. Rachel was willing to devote herself to getting rid of her disease, and she succeeded.

Two of the most dramatic successes I have had with arthritis came years later, when I had established my practice in San Francisco.

One of these was a beautiful, dark-haired woman named Eileen. She was in her mid-thirties when she was stricken with both asthma and rheumatoid arthritis. She was taking twelve aspirins a day for her constant, severe pain. A doctor who also practiced acupuncture had helped her overcome her asthma, but her arthritis was only getting worse and worse.

Eileen couldn't even button her blouse or get herself into and out of the bathtub. Her steps were slow and shuffling, and she deteriorated to the point where, frustrated by the pain and immobility, she became apathetic about everything, even her four-year-old son. She only wanted to lie still and be left alone. Her doctor told her she could expect only further deterioration.

Eileen had two friends who had been my patients, and they both tried to persuade her to see me, but she refused to consider it. Finally, the Roshi (head priest) of the Zen Buddhist community where she lived insisted on it, and she came to my office, depressed and pessimistic. Eileen was completely resistant and unwilling to change.

I told her during our first session that she would be completely cured of arthritis, but she did not believe me. The swelling and stiffness in her fingers, the constant pain in her toes, where the arthritis had started, the stiff, swollen ankles and knees, the immobile pelvis and rigid spine, congested chest, and unbearable pain in her neck and shoulders contradicted anything I could say. She was dragging her feet, hardly breathing, and hardly moving.

Within a month, Eileen and I reached an impasse. Her refusal to cooperate was very frustrating for me. I began to feel that she was more affected by her disease than she needed to be. It was as if she was cooperating with her arthritis in order to destroy herself. This made me extremely angry. When she dragged herself into my office for our sixth session, her walking was worse than ever. I told her to stand in the middle of the room and to lift her leg and rest it on a chair I had placed there. It took several minutes to do this, and her leg was shaking as if spastic. Then I asked her to do it with the other leg, and she had even more difficulty. Then I asked her to swing one leg up and over the back of the chair, and she did this very slowly, stopping to rest her foot on the seat of the chair on the way down.

When she finished doing this with the other leg, I could barely contain my fury, "If you can swing your leg over a chair that high, why can't you walk without dragging your feet? When I walk, I lift my knees. If I locked my knees and walked as you do, I'd have arthritis too. No wonder your cartilage is damaged. Stop dragging your feet!"

Eileen was visibly shaken at my tone. "Do you still think you can do something for me?" she asked.

"That depends on your willingness to cooperate. If you ever walk that way again, I will stop treating you."

After that session, Eileen began to work hard learning to walk without dragging her feet. She also began to reduce her aspirin intake, and the pain and swelling in her knees decreased. Although it was difficult, she began to lift her knees when she walked, easing the burden of pressure on them, and to coordinate her steps with the movement of her arms. Soon it was obvious that the swelling in her toes, ankles, knees, and hands was decreasing. Though she still felt discouraged, Eileen could see the improvement and could understand that she had to learn how to move correctly.

I instructed Eileen to move every joint of her body, including each joint of each finger and toe, in both lateral and rotating motions. At first this was very difficult for her to do without long sessions of massage, which she had twice a week. When working on her own, however, she would first breathe deeply for some minutes and visualize each joint moving, expanding as she inhaled and shrinking as she exhaled. Thus she worked both on her body and on her mental concept of her body. She would count 100 deep breaths, and with each she would "send" the oxygen to a different joint. She would work on the least afflicted joints first – the back, hips, elbows and hands – rotating, bending, opening and closing the hands. Her toes and ankles were the most severely afflicted, the first to show signs of damage, and they were the last things she should work on. One ankle was so weak she could actually walk better on it when it was swollen, using the swelling as support! To work on that ankle, she needed first to reduce the swelling, which she did by going to the beach and walking in the shallow water. The cold water not only reduced the swelling, but increased circulation to the area which made it easier for her to move it and so strengthen it.

As Eileen continued to improve, slowly but steadily, I continued to call her attention to many mistakes she was making in movement, from the way she walked to the way she put on and took off her coat. She had been using a few muscles very strenuously, and my criticism and teasing helped her realize this.

Eileen was very intelligent. She had a graduate degree in psychology and was studying Zen meditation. At the same time she felt many emotional conflicts. She carried a deep anger against her father, who had mistreated her as a child, and against the Zen Roshi who had become a father figure for her. She was torn between a wish to submit to a higher authority and a fierce independence and rebelliousness. This conflict left her paralyzed and affected even her immune system, causing her white blood cells to attack her cartilage and destroy it. This is the main characteristic that differentiates rheumatoid from osteoarthritis.

Eileen became increasingly annoyed by my criticisms. One

day when I began to tease her, instead of responding verbally as she usually did, she fought back physically. We began wrestling, and I made sure that every joint in her body moved. I lifted her on to the trampoline in our office and she kicked and punched me as hard as she could. In the process she was using her hips, knees, shoulders, and neck. Another patient who witnessed this said afterwards, "I'm not sure that fighting is therapeutic, but it is obvious that Eileen is much better afterwards." Eileen too appreciated the thera- peutic value of our "exercise," but she had been trying to beat me up. Fighting released some of her anger against me and transformed it into constructive energy. Increasingly, vitality returned to her, and she began to look more attractive and act more concerned about those around her. Even her attitude toward me relaxed, and I felt that it was time for her to begin to really work on herself.

On top of her double load as a working mother, Eileen began to do two hours of exercise every day, moving every joint in her body. She put all her anger into the exercises. Anger became the driving force in her life, and she really came alive. From extreme apathy, she came to have strong, vital feelings. One day while she was shopping, Eileen noticed that it was no great effort to carry her packages, and that awakened in her the realization that she was going to recover. She began to relax for the first time since she had become sick.

The next step for Eileen was using the trampoline to loosen her joints and overcome her fear of movement. A trampoline offers less resistance than ordinary ground, so that bouncing on it is almost effortless. At first Eileen was afraid of falling, so she sat and bounced on to her buttocks and then up on to her feet. Next she kneeled and bounced first on to her knees and then on to her feet. Each time she did this, she could walk more easily the next day.

Eileen's next step was to stop taking aspirin. She gradually decreased the dosage until she agreed to throw them away altogether. Soon after this she became depressed. She wondered why after all this improvement and increase in energy, she still suffered so much fatigue and pain. By giving up aspirin, she had taken her body out of its state of numbness, and the return of feeling made her believe she was getting worse, though experiencing her feelings of discomfort was actually an indication that she was getting better. Because for the first time she was able to feel how serious her condition was, she was temporarily overwhelmed by it.

Fortunately, only a few weeks after she stopped taking aspirin, Eileen was invited by her father to join him for a vacation in Acapulco. There she exercised every day on the beach in the warm sun and in the water, and began to feel completely renewed. Her father, who had not seen her for a year, was delighted with her improvement.

When she returned, Eileen quit her job and began to swim and exercise in a warm pool and to work on herself at home for four or more hours a day. She learned to work creatively and with a greater awareness of her body's needs. Exercises under water are designed for freer movement with less gravitational resistance. It is as if the body becomes a part of the water. Warm water relaxes and expands the body, and this elongates the muscles and creates more space between the bones. Exercises which are virtually impossible for an arthritic patient in ordinary circumstances become easy in water. Eileen was able to rotate her feet, open and close her hands, and even walk smoothly in warm water. In addition to the benefits of decreased gravitational resistance, water itself offers a constant, soft resistance which strengthens the muscles with minimal challenge.

Finally, two years after we had begun to work together, I told Eileen she no longer had arthritis. She didn't believe me; so I encouraged her to see her physician for a re-diagnosis. When the results of the blood test came back, her doctor confirmed that I was correct. Her arthritis was gone.

Eileen improved so much that she decided to study my work and become a practitioner herself. While she was still my patient, she worked on the other secretaries at her office and showed such a natural talent that she decided to enroll in my practitioner training course. Only a slight limp remained from her illness, and her enthusiasm for our work was so great that she began to address large groups on the subject of self-healing.

However, she still had not resolved her deepest problem, the conflict with her father. She once told me that she had left home in great anger and resentment, determined never to ask her parents for anything. She used all her cash to rent an apartment and get a job and for two weeks, as she waited for her paycheck, she had nothing to eat. One time she was invited out for lunch, and she ate so much that she had to excuse herself and run to the women's room to vomit. Her escort did not ask her out again.

Because she had never been able to win her father's approval, she never fully accepted herself either, and always managed to thwart herself when she was on the brink of a great achievement. She would work hard, achieve much, then back away, dissatisfied. The rage at her father had never been resolved, and Eileen decided it was time to sort things out. She stopped seeing patients for a while and devoted herself to her meditation and her Zen community. Her body continued to improve and her life was happy and full. Within a year, Eileen had married, and later was appointed secretarial assistant to the Roshi.

Then came a fresh disaster. The Roshi was accused of wrongdoing, and many in the community turned against him. From being an almost God-like figure, respected by the entire community, he suddenly became the focus of their fears, frustrations, and failings. They had expected so much from him that they could not tolerate his apparent shortcomings.

To Eileen, for whom the Roshi had taken a father's place in

her affection and respect, this situation created an unbearable conflict. She had a crippling attack, so severe that it took two years for her to recover from it. During that time I worked on her nearly every day. Even during my advanced training class in which she was a student, I would massage her ankle as I lectured.

I felt that a cleansing fast would help her, so Eileen and I went off for a six-day retreat in the Trinity Alps in California. We stayed in a cabin by a lake, and fasted on vegetable juices. I encouraged Eileen to talk for hours about her relationship with her father, and on the fifth day, she suddenly burst out, "I just can't see myself getting over this anger! I can't see myself getting strong enough to forgive my father, or Roshi. I can't see myself getting well!"

This outburst was very healthy. Eileen had been the victim of her own resentment for years, but had never before fully experienced it. Now she could experience her rage, not just in her muscles and joints, but in her conscious mind. I could not answer her with words; no words would have helped. But through massage and exercise Eileen began to cleanse herself emotionally, and at last she could forgive them.

From that time on her health improved rapidly. Eileen resumed her career as a self-healing practitioner, and she is one of the best.

I met Kristin shortly after she had undergone hip-replacement surgery. Like Eileen, Kristin had rheumatoid arthritis, but hers had progressed so rapidly that at age 25, the cartilage in both hips was gone. After an operation in which one worn-out hip joint was replaced with a plastic one, Kristin decided against further surgery. The operation and recovery had been so painful that she was given morphine as a pain killer, and she became addicted to it. Then she was given methadone as a substitute for the morphine, and became addicted to that instead.

Kristin knew about our Center before the operation, but

had decided in favor of the surgery. Her pain seemed such a waste to me; I was sure that she could have saved that hip.

Kristin was an angelically beautiful and frail young woman. Between pain, hospitalization, surgery, and medication, she had lost thirty pounds from an already slender frame. Her voice was almost a whisper. She leaned on a big black cane and on the arm of her brother, who had brought her to our office. Kristin could not walk without her cane, and her doctor was surprised that she could walk even with it.

Besides methadone, she was taking anti-inflammatory drugs. She had been given injections of cortisone as well, but these had no effect. Her disease showed in every joint in her body, but especially in her knees, where the swelling was so bad that her kneecaps were hidden beneath the accumulated fluid.

Kristin began our therapy with three sessions a week, each with a different practitioner. Her condition improved almost immediately. Kristin was rigid and stiff and extremely sensitive to cold. Her condition presented some unusual difficulties in the treatment. The removal of her hip joint made it very difficult for her to turn over; she had to be moved, and moved very gently. I usually had her lie on her side with the lower leg extended and the upper leg bent at the knee, to stretch out the hip. Then I would massage the buttock and outer thigh muscles gently with oil until they were warm. This increased the circulation not only to the hip but all over the body. I instructed her to lie and breathe, and be aware of her lower abdominal muscles as she did so, and I showed her how to massage her own hip, and strike it very gently with her fist. I had her lie on her back with bent knees and move the knees slowly from side to side, to activate the inner psoas muscles.

For the first six months she exercised two hours every day. Most of this was done lying down on her back, and its purpose was to bring circulation into the hip area without taxing the body or making an effort. I also showed her exercises to do in the bathtub, such as bending and straightening the knees and rotating the ankles. She liked to exercise in the sun, and as the only place she could do this was on the windy roof of the building where she lived, she soon learned to be comfortable with the cold breezes, and to accept variations in temperature more easily. She even started taking cold showers, which she now says make her feel better than anything else. Walking and dressing became easier for her and, encouraged by this, she began to work on herself for three to four hours a day. She felt stronger emotionally, and after a few months, decided to end her dependence on methadone. A hospital–run detoxification program helped her to accomplish this.

During a weekend workshop I gave, after two days of working and meditating on her body, Kristin found herself in tears, overwhelmed by emotions she could not understand. Those tears must have released something very deep inside her, for after that workshop, the swelling in her knees decreased considerably, and her kneecaps were visible for the first time in years.

As with Eileen, I took Kristin to exercise in a warm pool. The first time we went, I showed her what it was like to experience movement without resistance to gravity. When she got out of the pool, the sudden return of gravity was so jarring that she could only walk a few steps. At last she was aware of how she put effort and resistance into her every movement. This awareness, more than anything I could say, showed her what she needed to do.

After six months of therapy, Kristin could walk with her cane for four blocks. When I first met her she could barely cross the room! Her doctor in San Francisco – a student of her doctor in Los Angeles – was very impressed, saying, "Your X-rays show no cartilage in your hip joint. I don't understand how you can walk at all. Whatever it is you are doing, keep it up."

Within a year she was walking comfortably without her cane for short distances, and within two years, she was able to walk *one mile*. She joyfully reported each new breakthrough – the day she could sit down on the floor and get up again without help, and the wonderful day she could get into and out of the bathtub by herself. She stopped using anti-inflammatory drugs and now took only vitamins.

Two years after she began therapy with us, Kristin returned to Los Angeles to visit her doctor, a leading rheumatologist. At his urging, new X-rays were taken, and when they came back, the results were astonishing. Where former X-rays had shown no cartilage and no space between the bones and the hip joint, there was now a clearly visible space. Only seven cases like this are recorded in medical history. Her doctor showed these findings to a group of rheumatologists, none of whom could understand the change, but all agreed that a great improvement had indeed taken place. Those X-rays were an absolute triumph. I had not needed them to confirm Kristin's improvement; I could see it and feel it. But the X-rays served as proof that such an improvement can happen.

I flew to Los Angeles to meet with Kristin's doctor, and he agreed that self-healing exercises had been in great part responsible for Kristin's improvement. He was not convinced, however, that the space in the hip joint was created by regenerated cartilage, and was not ready to believe that cartilage could regenerate at all. Medical opinion stands firmly against this idea, but I have always been convinced that any body tissue can regenerate, given the right conditions. Kristin stands as living proof that even the most severe forms of arthritis can be overcome.

Chapter 10

Multiple sclerosis

Multiple sclerosis is a disease of the central nervous system in which the myelin sheath, the fatty tissue which protects the nerves, begins to break down, making it difficult for messages to be transmitted between the brain and the rest of the body. This disease is considered incurable, but based on results from our own therapy, I know it is possible for sufferers from multiple sclerosis to reach a level of remission that can be considered a cure. Multiple sclerosis attacks often come in waves, and are generally the result of a shock of some kind. It is not known what causes multiple sclerosis. There are two major medical theories. One, which is losing popularity, suggests that multiple sclerosis is caused by a virus which somehow inhibits the production of the myelin sheath. A more recent theory says that it may be caused by a breakdown of the immune system, which would allow viruses to attack the myelin sheath.

In my opinion, multiple sclerosis is related to an overload of the central nervous system due to overusing some neural pathways and underusing others. This is a result of stiff and unbalanced use of the body. A typical multiple sclerosis patient has poor posture and a rigid spine. She moves as if her body's center is in her neck, which puts a great strain there. Her back is so tense that not only the back muscles but also the viscera are constricted. And her whole body is so tight that even her walk is affected. Such extreme tension of muscles and organs leads to neurological dysfunction. The disappearance of parts of the myelin sheath is not the cause of multiple sclerosis, but is simply one of the worst symptoms, a result of misusing the body.

Ilana came to see me at the Vegetarian Society when she was in the early stages of multiple sclerosis. She walked unsteadily, with a limp, and her hips appeared to be unbalanced. She experienced numbness in various parts of her body, and this sometimes caused her to lose control of her bladder. A public school teacher, Ilana was afraid she might lose her job as a result of her illness.

I went to work on her right hand and arm which were partially paralyzed. The muscles she could still use were extremely sore from strained overuse. I taught Ilana a few simple exercises for the arm and worked with her to improve her breathing. Ilana expressed skepticism that any treatment could help her, but as she dressed after the treatment she found that she was able to button her blouse with no trouble – something she had been unable to do for months. Her arm felt lighter, with more sensation. Since she was doubtful, I suggested she try just three more treatments, to see if they were useful. She agreed, saying, "What have I got to lose?"

I gave Ilana some exercises for her lower back, which was extremely weak and tense. I had her lie on her back with her knees bent, her hands over her chest, and her head on a firm pillow so that her neck could relax. At first, it was difficult for her to keep her knees in this position for more than a few seconds, but after three weeks, she could do it for fifteen minutes. I asked her to breathe deeply and count the length of each inhalation and exhalation to help her concentrate on her breath and keep her mind off her knees, and to send thoughts of relaxation and expansion into her lower back, imagining it growing wider and longer. Her hips were tight and her ankles stiff, so I asked her to lie in a bathtub and bend and straighten her knees, and then move her feet one by one in rotating motion to strengthen the ankles and increase her balance. I also gave her many visualization exercises to help her sense how she used her body – how she moved her arms and legs as though they were extremely heavy, for example, and how her whole body would contract in order to perform one small movement. I wanted to reprogram her nervous system so that it would allow each muscle to do its own work.

Ilana was astonished at the number of changes which occurred during the sessions. Her pelvis loosened up. Though it was still difficult for her to walk, she could easily lift her legs to put on her shoes. She went swimming after our third session and could hardly believe that although a few weeks earlier she could barely swim a few yards, she now found herself swimming the length of the pool twice. Amazed at the changes she had experienced so quickly, Ilana consulted her doctor, who confirmed the improvement and encouraged her to continue.

After six weeks, Ilana could lie on her back with her knees bent for half an hour. She even once fell asleep in that position. Her earlier difficulty had come from tensing her knees and ankles. Once Ilana's back had released its tension, it was free to support itself. Her legs no longer had to work to support it, or have their own movement restricted by the lower back's tightness.

Although the muscles Ilana was now using had been weak from disuse, they grew stronger as she began using them in a correct and healthy way. Most importantly, she was changing old ingrained neurological patterns and her brain's belief that her back was weak and her legs immobile. Her doctor continued to confirm that her knee was getting stronger, and that her walk and reflexes were improving. This, along with small discoveries on her own – for example, she could sew for the first time in years – convinced Ilana to return to work in the fall.

Bladder weakness is common among multiple sclerosis patients. The need to urinate is unbearably urgent and difficult to control. Visualization and sphincter control exercises proved invaluable in treating this. I instructed Ilana to contract her bladder muscles as tightly as she could, while imagining that she was holding in urine forcibly, and to contract her upper body as tightly as possible, including the eyes and mouth, and to forcibly expel her breath through her teeth. Then, alternately, she would bear down on the bladder as if she were trying to expel urine but couldn't. This exercise helped Ilana achieve control of her bladder, and I have given it to every patient since who complained of lack of bladder control.

Vered, who is very observant about character and human nature, noticed Ilana's rigidity of mind. Although she was an intelligent and educated woman with many interests, Ilana had inexplicable mental blocks. For example, she was a teacher, but she never completely learned Hebrew, and continued certain foreign speech patterns which sounded comical in Hebrew. It was as if some parts of her mind were not in communication with the rest of it. She spoke in a dogmatic way, and gave the impression of inflexibility of mind and body.

Then, as if by magic, when her body learned to relax and trust her mind followed suit. She became open to more possibilities, including the possibility of a cure for her illness. Her new attitude seemed to grow naturally out of her new experiences with her body.

I worked with Ilana until I left Israel, and in all that time she did not experience any further degeneration. She never completely lost her limp, but it diminished and her balance improved dramatically. She regained the coordination in her hands, and her mental state continued to improve, as she gained trust in herself. It was Ilana who gave me confidence that multiple sclerosis, although an extraordinary challenge, was something we could help.

Sophia Gefen was referred to us by another patient, Hannah. As the wife of an orthodox Rabbi, Sophia was the teacher for the women of the synagogue. Her husband, a kind and simple man, had done all he could to make her life easier after she was stricken with multiple sclerosis, and he felt much grief about her illness. He drove her around to doctors and helped her with errands and household chores. It was obvious that Sophia was deeply loved and respected by everyone who knew her.

The first symptom she had experienced was a lack of sensation in her hands and feet. When she washed dishes, they would often slip out of her hands without her feeling it. Her hands were so lacking in sensation that she did not even experience numbness. She felt that her hands were immobile and clenched, even when they were open. She realized she had the same problem with her feet when one day she arrived home after shopping and found that she had lost her shoes in the street while walking, and hadn't even noticed it. Tests at the neurology clinic of her hospital were performed by stabbing her hands and feet with sharp objects to the point of bleeding, and she still felt no pain. The doctors confirmed Sophia's worst fears when they told her she had multiple sclerosis.

She was hospitalized and given drugs, but her condition did not improve, and she was released. She and her husband asked her neurologist, "Is there anything in the world we can do?" He replied kindly, "There is nothing medical I know of that will help. Sophia will probably come to see me every six months with another attack and will steadily deteriorate. But don't give up," he added with concern. "You should pray. There is always hope."

From that time on, Sophia was hospitalized every two or three months. Although her attacks gradually decreased in frequency, they increased in severity, and she had no remission or improvement. In cases of multiple sclerosis, there is usually a remission period after an attack, during which the patient experiences some improvement. Sometimes the effects of the attack almost disappear. But Sophia's symptoms only worsened. When her physicians saw no improvement over a long period of time, they rediagnosed her illness as amyotrophic lateral sclerosis (ALS), commonly known as Lou Gehrig's disease, in which there are no remissions. ALS causes the patient to deteriorate much more rapidly than multiple sclerosis.

As her condition continued to worsen, the diagnosis was confirmed. Sophia's balance and coordination almost disappeared, and she was on the verge of paralysis. She could no longer perform any tasks which required hand coordination. Her walking was slow and heavy, when she was able to walk at all. At most, she could walk only the length of her room. Her doctors told her husband that Sophia had no more than eighteen months to live.

A discouraging prognosis handed down by a trusted physician may hasten a patient's death. We have become entirely dependent on doctors for information about our own bodies, our diseases, and hope for recovery. Physicians should use this awesome power carefully, to help encourage their patients rather than exacerbate their fears. Patients should always be encouraged to keep up hope and to seek every possible solution to a problem. No one should be given an absolutely hopeless prognosis, for this may become a self-fulfilling prophecy. Patients should not treat a physician's prognosis as the only possible outcome.

Sophia's husband and children accompanied her to her first meeting with me and were present for our session. Sophia walked in as if her feet were too heavy to lift. She could barely hold herself upright, much less drag herself across the room. Her expression was one of fear, and it seemed to me that this fear was a big part of her difficulty in walking. She seemed to be afraid of each step she took. She would raise one foot just barely off the floor, tensing her whole body, even her face, and then she would throw her entire weight on to that foot and drag the other one after it. After a few steps, she needed to collapse or grab something for support. What she feared most was losing her balance. Without realizing it, she was hardly breathing, and the few breaths she took were through her mouth. Her energy seemed almost nonexistent.

I helped Sophia on to the table and asked her to lie on her back. Then, with her knees bent and her feet flat on the table, I started to teach her breathing exercises. As is often the case with severely injured or crippled patients, she needed to learn breathing first. I asked her to inhale deeply and slowly, then to exhale completely and to wait as long as she could, about twenty seconds, before breathing again, and to repeat the whole process. She did this about one hundred times.

Sophia began to feel her body with which she had become completely out of touch. The first sensation she experienced was extreme heaviness. She was convinced that the session had helped her, but her husband and children were skeptical, so she decided not to continue the treatment. When Hannah heard about this, she visited Sophia repeatedly and finally convinced her to continue my treatment in earnest. After an interim of two months, Sophia came to my office again. She remembered the exercises I had shown her, and after a couple of weeks of small improvements, she said to me, "Meir, this treatment is a great encouragement."

I said, "I hope the effects are not just psychological."

She answered, "No, I am feeling much better, both psychologically and physically, and it gives me hope."

About a month later, it became obvious to everyone that her state of mind and body was better. Before this, she had wanted to do nothing. Now she wanted to be involved in as many activities as she could. She was more interested in her condition and willing to devote herself to her recovery. Even her family began to believe it might be possible.

Sophia's husband was under a great deal of stress because of her condition. Sometimes when he brought her to see me I would massage his shoulders and neck. One time I even stood with him back to back, took hold of his arms, and bent forward until I was holding him off the floor on my back. Sophia was amazed to see this, as he was much taller and heavier than I was. While supporting him in this way, I stretched his arms, neck, shoulders, and back by pulling gently on his arms. This released a lot of his tension, and he was able to sit and relax as he watched our session.

Within two months, Sophia's balance was noticeably better. Although not consistent or reliable, she had less tendency to fall. She also had a few hours of relief each day from her constant fatigue. One day Sophia said, "I feel that something wonderful is about to happen to me." She could foresee a great change. Sometimes when patients talk about the improvement they expect, they are engaging in wishful thinking. Once in a while, someone will speak about his or her improvement with conviction based on deep inner knowledge. When Sophia said that a great change for the better would take place in her life, I sensed that she was right.

From that time on, Sophia's therapy was entirely different. It wasn't Danny, Vered and I working to give Sophia back her health. We just assisted her. The four of us were working together.

Within a month, Sophia began to come to our sessions on her own. She could get on and off the bus and walk from the bus stop to our office. Her step was becoming noticeably lighter, although she still limped. Walking did not tire her nearly as much as it had. She felt a renewed sense of enthusiasm, and she began to take walks every day. Her improvements reaffirmed her hope for a cure.

Sophia's coordination was still a big problem. Many simple tasks were difficult for her, and her movements were clumsy and ineffectual. Danny and Vered worked on her until her muscles were relaxed, and I concentrated on exercises. As a result, Sophia's breath became deeper and more regular, and the increased blood flow allowed her to perform movements which would otherwise have been difficult or even harmful.

After a while, Sophia came to understand how she tensed her body. By experiencing her body as relaxed sometimes, she became aware of the contrast. She could now work on moving with minimal strain. When we massaged Sophia's feet, it took her half an hour before she could move her ankle in a rotating motion without tensing her legs, back, chest, and stomach. In a short time, her calf muscles, some of which had been hard as steel from the tension of overworking, began to loosen. The calf muscles which had been completely unused and had deteriorated, began to slowly build up. This allowed her to stand more solidly on her feet, but did not completely solve her balance problem. I asked Sophia to stand on one foot. She began to fall over, but I caught her. We spent hours on this before she was able to stand on one foot even for a few seconds. Having done so, she found it a little easier to stay upright on two feet.

Danny, Vered, and I also worked on other parts of her body. Her hips were very tight and this caused a great deal of restriction in walking, so I instructed her to stand on both feet and move her pelvis in a rotating motion. Although for most people this is a simple motion, Sophia found it nearly impossible. She swung her hips in jerky, angular motions, rather than circles. Vered, who had a lot of experience with this exercise, showed her how to begin by making small circles and gradually increase the range of movement. She had Sophia tilt her pelvis forward, backward, right and left. In time Sophia learned to feel how much she could tilt without falling. Her balance began to improve and her hips became much looser. She began to feel more confident while walking.

Just as Danny, Vered, and I had done, Sophia began to

work on herself with near-fanatic zeal. She exercised for hours every day and she came to see us three times a week. While she lay on the table, one of us would take her arm or leg and gently stretch it, telling her to imagine that the limb stretched the length of the room, the length of the street, and finally stretching into infinity. We did this with each limb, and she felt as if her body expanded farther every time. As we stretched her limbs, we lengthened the muscles, and this allowed them to relax. Tense muscles are shorter, and lengthening the muscles allows more circulation, since the muscles don't then constrict the blood vessels. This feeling of expansion was very relaxing for Sophia and made her feel lighter and more open. In her imagery her body seemed to lose its boundaries. The restrictions which tension had imposed on her body seemed to dissolve.

The change in Sophia's conception of her body and its abilities led to a change in her conception of herself. Just as her body expanded and became capable of more and more, so, she felt, did she herself. In less than half a year, Sophia became an entirely different person. She wanted to learn new things, expand her narrow horizons, and change. She was especially eager to learn whatever she could from us. Sophia was a pleasure to work with. When we would show her an exercise which was very difficult at first, she would practice it at home and two days later show us that she had mastered it. Our sessions were a mutually beneficial exchange.

Although Sophia didn't exhibit any symptoms of damage to her optic nerve, I thought she might be vulnerable to eye problems since these are common to the multiple sclerosis family of diseases. A person can have an inherent tendency towards a problem without showing any symptoms, so rather than wait for this symptom to manifest itself, I decided to offer preventative therapy. I showed her palming and sunning and other exercises. She would get headaches after doing them, but I explained that this was common for someone just beginning to do them. The muscular relaxation gained makes one more aware of previously unnoticed tensions around the eyes. These tensions, along with increased stimulation of the optic nerve, were partially responsible for the headaches. The headaches, therefore, were a sign that the nerves needed to be stimulated and relaxed, and that it had been a good idea for her to do eye exercises. I showed Sophia how to massage her head and face to relieve the headaches, but there was a lot of work to do to awaken and heal the degenerated optic nerve. It took Sophia eighteen months before she could do eye exercises daily, in comfort.

Sophia and her husband took walks together every evening, and when they reached a mile, he was more tired than she. After only six months, most of her symptoms had disappeared. Only one major symptom remained: Sophia still could feel nothing in her hands and feet. I called Dr Arkin, who was an associate of Sophia's neurologist, and he said there was nothing that could be done to restore her sensation. He had studied her case and the damage was in her central nervous system. He felt nothing could be done to repair it. "There has been no case of ALS or multiple sclerosis to my knowledge where sensation has returned," he said, "so please just be grateful for what an excellent job you have done." I was not convinced that Dr Arkin was right. I felt that if anyone deserved health it was Sophia. She had worked hard on herself and was doing everything she could to get well.

I started to rub Sophia's fingers every time she came to see me, putting all my love and faith into each massage. I used hand cream to warm her skin and reduce the friction of massage. Each time I would ask her, "Can you feel anything now?" and she would answer, "No, not a thing."

Finally one evening, in despair, I called Miriam. I described Sophia's condition, and after asking a few questions Miriam understood the whole picture. Then she asked me, "You know what to do in a case like this, don't you?"

"Would I ask you if I knew?" I answered impatiently.

Ignoring me, Miriam continued, "It's so simple. All you need to do is tell her to tap her fingers on a table."

I was astonished. It really was simple. Why hadn't I thought of that? I was certain that Sophia would be able to feel with her hands. I didn't understand the effect such an exercise would have, but it was clear to me that the stimulation of the nerve endings that would be produced by this exercise would have an influence on the central nervous system.

Sophia came to see me for her next appointment on a Friday morning, ready to face a hectic day of preparations and then a restful Sabbath. She was surprised when I asked her to sit down at my desk rather than go into the treatment room, and I sat down beside her. I experienced a kind of mental union with Sophia at that moment, so complete was my empathy with her.

As Miriam suggested, I told Sophia to tap her fingertips on the desk top. She responded without hesitation, tapping quickly and rhythmically. I sensed that this caused her some pain, and she confirmed that this was so. The pain diminished after tapping for about fifty times, and then disappeared. After tapping about one hundred times, she began to sense pressure in her fingertips. She continued the tapping and gradually the pressure also disappeared and she felt only numbness – this was after she had tapped about three hundred times. I did the exercise with her, and to my astonishment, it was as if I felt each of her feelings in my own body. By the time we reached seven hundred, there was no pain and no pressure, only a continuous feeling of stimulation.

I told Sophia to breathe deeply and relax her shoulders, so that we could continue the exercise as long as possible. After tapping a thousand times, her hands felt as if they were capable of complete, normal sensation.

We started to tap on the knuckles nearest the fingertips and had the same experience that we had had with the fingertips, except that it took only half as long to achieve the same results. When the pain came, it was a strong sensation, not numb or distant. Then we repeated the exercise with the middle knuckles with similar results, but with an increased level of sensation, pressure, and pain. Once the process of awakening had begun, it was almost instantaneous. We tapped very gently at first, slowly increasing the intensity.

Finally we worked on the largest knuckles, those where the fingers connect to the hand, and it followed the same progression, through numbness to pain to painless pressure to tingling. Then we began to tap on the table with our outer wrist joints. By this time Sophia was able to feel everything that she touched, and her hands no longer felt clenched and locked, as they had for months. They actually felt relaxed.

I let Sophia lie down on the table and I massaged her for a while. Then I began to test her. I gave her a pen, and she was able to identify it just by touching it. I gave her a pencil and she identified it as a pencil and not a pen, because she was able to feel that it was made of wood. I called Danny and Vered in to share in our triumph. I was so happy I was in tears. Sophia's was the greatest improvement I had seen. For both Sophia and me, this was the happiest day of our lives.

For the next few weeks, we used the same exercise to help restore sensation in Sophia's feet. It took longer to accomplish this than with her fingers. Sophia couldn't raise her legs easily, so we assisted her in tapping with her feet. But after three weeks, she began to feel something in her heels, and with a lot of exercise and massage, some, though not all, feeling was regained.

I called Miriam to tell her about Sophia's success and she took the news quite calmly. The results were as she had expected.

Then with great excitement, I called Dr Arkin. He was incredulous and even defensive at first, but soon he was convinced that I was telling the truth. When he saw Sophia a few weeks later, he was amazed. As a result, he began to refer other neurological patients to us.

The doctors at Sophia's hospital had a different reaction. When they saw Sophia's vast improvement, they changed their diagnosis back from ALS to multiple sclerosis, and called the improvement a remission. They overlooked that even in MS, no patient has been known to have remission from a prolonged and total lack of sensation. We are not talking about numbness, which is itself a sensation, but about a total lack of feeling.

I cannot claim a cure, *per se*, for MS or ALS. But I can offer the possibility of health for anyone willing to invest the time and effort. Sophia was such a person. She determined to cure herself and she succeeded. She thoroughly earned that cure. Sophia had no preconceptions or prejudices; she did not approach the matter intellectually. She just proceeded with confidence and trust that something would happen. With such an attitude, any disease can be overcome.

A short time later, Dr Arkin referred Menachem, a restaurant owner, to us. Menachem had been hospitalized frequently with multiple sclerosis attacks, and he was overcome with despair. He spent two weeks in the hospital unable to lie, sit, or stand without feeling dizzy. When he was released, still suffering from dizziness, he went to the hospital's neurology department where the five neurology specialists were having a meeting. He interrupted them to tell his story, and asked, "Is there anything you can do for me?" They all shook their heads. So Menachem left, but waited outside by the door, and as the neurologists left the meeting, he asked each of them one by one, "Can you help me?" and each one repeated, "No, I'm sorry." But Dr Arkin added, "I know of no cure for MS, but I can give you an unofficial referral to some people who have had some success with it. I am not referring you to these people in my capacity as a doctor – this is strictly off the record." Dr Arkin was very cautious, and he made it clear that he could promise nothing.

So Menachem came to us as his last resort. I understood Dr Arkin's pessimism as soon as I started to test Menachem. His legs were so weak that he could barely stand up. A muscle test had shown that his leg muscles were almost nonfunctional. His limbs felt very heavy, both to him and to us. Danny commented that the more alive a person is, the lighter his limbs feel, and this feeling of heaviness is a kind of death. The sensation of heaviness has nothing to do with actual weight, Vered added.

If Menachem so much as turned his head to one side, he would lose his balance and fall. He walked like a drunk, swinging his whole body from side to side. He was constantly fatigued, and simply seemed tired of life. He could see no sense in doing anything, when every movement brought with it a bout of dizziness, often accompanied by nausea.

At first we had no idea what to do. No medical answers had been found. Doctors had tried giving him cortisone, and sometimes vitamin B–12, but these had not succeeded. Even in his remissions from MS, his dizziness continued to worsen every day.

Menachem's wife had left him because of his illness, and his children came to see him only occasionally. He had been forced to lease his restaurant because he couldn't run it by himself. He was about to sell his house and go to live with his parents, and had only delayed doing it because he did not have the physical or emotional strength to put the house on the market.

During our first meeting with Menachem, I told him that we expected him to do a number of exercises. I could feel his reluctance to do anything. It was not only the strain and discomfort that any action caused him, it was also that his body needed a lot of rest. We decided to see Menachem three times a week. The first thing I did with him was to slowly and gently move each of his limbs, to encourage circulation. We also went to work on his eye problems. His optic nerve had degenerated and his vision was blurred. Palming helped a great deal. Not only did it give his eyes some relief, but through resting his eyes he was able to relax his whole body. He became aware of a feeling that something was constantly choking him from within, emotionally and physically, and this feeling was released when he palmed.

After only two weeks, Menachem's walking began to show signs of improvement. We had instructed him to move his feet in a rotating motion several hundred times a day, and as a result his calves were stronger. Feeling more relaxed increased his confidence and his constant fear of falling was alleviated. Still, the way Menachem walked was not very good. He limped, and it was difficult for him to raise his legs. During our seventh session, Menachem told me, "I'm starting to get better. I'm still dizzy and I am still limping, but I feel better inside. I feel like I want to do things." He told me that the day before, he had gone to his restaurant and asked the people leasing it to let him do some work there. He had felt dizzy, but he worked for two hours. "I'm tired of staying in bed," he confided. This improvement touched me deeply. I felt a change in his state of mind, and I believed he was going to succeed.

Menachem still had ups and downs. At one session he told Vered he didn't know how he could continue to live with constant dizziness. But his new hope could meet that despair. It was during that session with Vered while she was massaging the back of his head, that he experienced his first temporary relief from dizziness. Though this reprieve only lasted a few hours, it was a sign that the condition could be relieved.

Miriam once told me that she had suffered from severe headaches for many years. One had been so extreme that she could not do anything. In the midst of it, she lay down on the floor and began to move her head in slow rotations. At first the pain increased even more, and she felt as if her whole body would explode, but she continued to rotate her head while massaging her scalp. Within thirty minutes the headache passed, and she has never had another one.

This is like piling blankets on a fever patient to help her "sweat out" the fever. The symptom is encouraged to reach a peak level so that it can pass more quickly. This is in the spirit of the fundamental principal of homeopathy. It occurred to me that Menachem's problem might be treated a similar way.

After two and a half months of working with Menachem, when he arrived at our office suffering as much as ever from dizziness, I asked him to stand in front of the window and move his head in a rotating motion. "I can't possibly do that," he protested. "I'm dizzy enough as it is." But I insisted, and for some reason he trusted me enough to try it. He completed one circular motion and became nauseated. He tried again and grew even sicker, with a suffocating sensation in his solar plexus. On the third try he thought he would vomit, and on the fourth try he did. His face turned a pale yellow-green and he said, "I'm going to faint." His body was cold and moist, so I helped him onto the table and rubbed him with oil to warm him. I massaged him until he was warm again, the nausea had passed, and his skin was rosy.

We went out on the porch and tried again. He felt weak and sick, but this time he was able to move his head seven times around before he became pale and chilled, and vomited again. I took him back to the table for another massage.

We did this a third time with the same results. I could hardly believe either of us was willing to continue, but somehow we both felt we were doing the right thing. After the fourth try, Menachem began to have less trouble with the exercise. His circulation was becoming better and creating a more even distribution of blood between his head and his body.

All in all we repeated this exercise ten times! Each time it seemed to affect him a little less. The tenth time, I led him to the porch and he was able to move his head thirty times around in each direction. He told me, "I am not dizzy and I don't feel sick, but I am so weak and tired." We agreed that this was enough for one day. I massaged him once more, and instructed him not to eat anything for the rest of the day, and called a cab to take him home.

Menachem began to do this exercise daily. From the very next day, he was able to move his head in rotating motion two hundred times in each direction without becoming dizzy. From that time on, he improved dramatically. He could walk down the street and turn his head from side to side to look at the store windows. He could ride a bicycle for half an hour and could even jog a little.

Having been granted relief from his worst problem, Menachem began to get in touch with other aspects of his illness. He could now feel how weak and stiff his movements were, and how imbalanced his standing and walking. This new awareness changed Menachem's whole approach to life. No longer a hopeless victim of a mysterious ailment, he could now look at the cause of his problems and make an effort to effect a change.

Working with Menachem taught me much about the importance of centering in treating MS. After we had helped him overcome his dizziness and regain his balance, we had to help him restructure his entire habitual pattern of movement, especially walking, and help him to rebuild the muscles in his legs and feet.

Menachem's center was in the back of his head where it joins the neck, making it difficult for him to breathe deeply. This was indicated by the tension there, and by the fact that he threw his entire weight on his toes when he walked. I asked him to stand up straight and keep his feet parallel when he stood or walked and to concentrate on his body's center. I instructed him to breathe deeply into his abdomen to increase his awareness of that area, so that he could begin to re-focus his center of movement there, where it belonged. This exercise of "centering" helps people to become aware of where the force or impetus behind a movement or action comes from. This is not esoteric knowledge – anyone who pays attention to his body can learn to "center." A sensation of lightness flowed through him as he breathed. I then placed my hands on his abdomen and asked him to visualize that his back was relaxing, growing wider and longer. When I did this, Menachem experienced a great release from his neck tension and could move his neck from side to side with no restriction, further than he had ever been able to before. As he continued this exercise – moving his head from side to side and visualizing his back growing wider and stronger, his neck lengthening, the top of his head going up to the sky, and his energy flowing from his center – Menachem's thoracic vertebrae began to make a popping sound, although I wasn't even touching them. This is a sign that his spine was lengthening and relaxing.

We then tried to incorporate this new awareness into his walking. Menachem's inclination was to return to his unbalanced, constricted walk. I coached him, reminding him to concentrate on his center and feel his back expanding, his shoulders extending, and his neck lengthening.

I then asked Menachem to sit and then rise without using his arms to help. This was very difficult for someone whose leg muscles were so tight as to be nearly paralyzed. He had come to the point where he no longer sat down but just collapsed into a chair and then used his arms to push himself up. Stretching and exercising his thigh muscles and maintaining an awareness of his abdominal center as the focal point of movement enabled Menachem to sit and rise in a coordinated and relaxed way.

I feel that it is much more important to discover why certain people develop MS symptoms and how they can be helped. Our work with Ilana, Sophia, Menachem and more than one hundred other MS patients reveals once again that no disease is incurable. All that is necessary is to take the time to study the individual's symptoms and the process that brings them about so we can change it from a process which encourages constriction to one which enhances movement, and therefore life.

Chapter 11

Breathing and visualization

Mr Solano heard me lecture at the Vegetarian Society. He had no serious malady but felt that he wanted to use his minor, ordinary problems as a way to learn about himself. A handsome man in his late forties, Mr Solano told me he had a very minor back problem and was often tired. He was a very open-minded, inquisitive man.

He had developed some tightness in his lower back as a result of poor posture and poor walking habits. Instead of putting his weight equally on each foot and equally on each part of the foot, he tended to land heavily on his right heel, which created pressure in his lower back. He also had occasional headaches. He wasn't especially concerned about his spine problem becoming more serious, but he felt that if he could learn to relax his spine, he would be able to relax his whole body, and as a result eliminate the headaches.

Not surprisingly, the treatment we found most effective for Mr Solano was to regulate and deepen his breathing. Shallow breathing causes constriction of every part of the body. With less oxygen coming in, all functioning becomes more difficult, one's energy level drops, and fatigue sets in. The heart is particularly affected, since the working of the lungs and heart are so closely connected.

If there is more oxygen in the body because of deeper breathing, the heart does not have to strain to pump blood to and from the rest of the body. Every cell in the body requires fresh oxygen as its fuel, and this is carried to each cell by the flow of blood. Veins carry de-oxygenated blood into the heart and the heart pumps it into the lungs, where it is enriched with oxygen. The blood then returns to the heart from where it is pumped through the arteries to the cells. If you do not breathe deeply enough and take in sufficient oxygen, the blood will leave the lungs without enough oxygen to adequately nourish the cells. The cells will then need to send the blood back for oxygen more frequently, requiring the heart to pump more than would be necessary if proper breathing had supplied enough oxygen to the lungs in the first place. With chronic shallow breathing, the cells are not adequately nourished, and one begins to feel fatigued. After a while, the cells become accustomed to this and do not even demand more oxygen. Fatigue, low energy, depression, and many common problems become a way of life. We no longer recognize them as problems – but they leave us more vulnerable to illness.

The way we breathe has an effect on our emotional lives. Fear, anger, and other negative emotions lose some of their impact when we breathe deeply, slowly, and regularly. Deep breathing brings with it a sense of peace and harmony. Breath is life, and the more slowly and deeply you breathe the more alive you are.

I asked Mr Solano to inhale and hold his breath for a count of sixty, then exhale and count to sixty before inhaling again, and to repeat this exercise ten times in a relaxed manner akin to meditation. It took him several weeks to work up to a count of sixty. To do this we had to work, through massage and exercise, on his diaphragm, chest, and stomach muscles, all of which are involved in deep breathing. This exercise encourages the patient to enjoy as fully as possible the benefits of oxygen. It creates a feeling in the body quite different from that created by rapid, shallow breathing.

I asked Mr Solano to visualize his breath as a breeze

blowing down into his abdomen, then up his spine, and into the back of his neck. I also asked him to describe what his breath sounded like, to encourage him to really listen to the sound and to experience deep relaxation. As Mr Solano was lying down, listening to his breath, he suddenly got quite cold. It was 90° Fahrenheit, a warm summer afternoon, and yet he was trembling. We were both startled, and Mr Solano asked me why he was feeling so cold. I thought for awhile, and the answer came, "You must be deeply relaxed." He responded, still shivering, "Yes, I am. In fact, I feel more relaxed and comfortable than ever." I have since observed that this commonly occurs during full relaxation. Since the central nervous system works to its fullest extent when the body feels chilled and slows down when the body is warm, and since relaxation *also* allows the central nervous system to function at its fullest extent, the body may associate relaxation with a sense of cooling off or an actual chill.

From that time on Mr Solano felt increasingly relaxed and expansive from within. He became so relaxed, in fact, that he set a new standard of relaxation for me. He stood evenly balanced on both feet. The tension which had controlled his mind and body for thirty years, which had brought on headaches, backaches, and a perpetual state of impatience and frustration, completely dissolved. Simple breathing exercises practiced for less than a month cured him of all these problems, and his general attitude about himself improved immensely.

At about the same time I began to work with a patient suffering from a type of anemia in which her body's supply of red blood cells had become depleted. (This is only one of many different types of anemia, but it is one of the most common.) Red blood cells, also called hemoglobin, are produced in the marrow of certain bones, such as the sternum, vertebrae, and others, or, in some cases of extreme hemoglobin, insufficiency in the liver and spleen. Through movement, breathing and bodywork, we can help to improve circulation and promote the normal hemoglobin-producing activity of the bone marrow.

Viva was a short, thin woman whose face was pale from lack of circulation. The skin on her palms and the soles of her feet was tough and rigid, and she suffered from eczema. She was constantly fatigued, and when she came to my office at the Vegetarian Society, she looked completely exhausted.

Viva was in her mid-thirties, the wife of a bus driver and the mother of two small children. Her parents were still so deeply involved in her life that she didn't know how to free herself from their influence. Viva felt completely oppressed by her circumstances. She felt she had no control of her life or her decisions.

Physicians tend to view anemia solely in terms of blood chemistry and treat it accordingly, but I think it should be viewed in terms of circulation. Inadequate circulation leads to deficiency in chemical composition. I knew that stimulating Viva's circulation would stimulate the organs responsible for the production of red blood cells.

I had two main objectives in my treatment of Viva. First I wanted to create good, strong circulation throughout her body. Second, I wanted to strengthen and relax her completely exhausted body. I told Viva to take alternating hot and cold showers. Warm water brings the circulation to the surface, relaxing the muscles, and cold water sends the blood deeper into the body's tissues, stimulating the internal organs and making the blood run faster to maintain the body's warmth. By relaxing her hips and shoulders with gentle exercise, and by massaging her hands and feet, we increased her circulation by drawing blood into the extremities, and thus made it flow strongly throughout the entire body. This, along with the application of a moisturizing cream, helped her eczema. I taught her deep breathing, which is extremely helpful to circulation, enriching the blood with oxygen. We used very few other movements at first. It was more helpful for her simply to lie and breathe. I was careful that she did not expend effort in breathing, for even breathing was an exertion for her and it was hard for her to learn to do it without straining.

Then we went on to small movements to reduce the stiffness in her muscles and joints, a condition which often accompanies anemia. I massaged her entire body, especially her cold, pale hands and feet. Her hands had a greenish tint and her feet were almost orange, but after massage both were a normal pinkish color. I worked a lot on her chest. It is in the muscles of the chest that negative emotions are often stored. I taught Viva to rub her hands together and then to rub her feet together while holding onto her calves. This was particularly difficult for her, and she grew tired almost immediately. In order to rub her feet together, she used her back, shoulders, and stomach with great effort. When she learned to relax the muscles which aren't needed for this movement, this exercise became very helpful for her, and she would do it continually until her feet became warm.

I showed Viva several different ways to massage her hands. With her fingers together and hands held straight, she would rub her hands together around 100 times. Then she would rub only the fingertips against each other, and then only the palms, in circular motions. The most effective variation was "hand washing," in which she would rub her hands and fingers together as if they were being lathered with soap. This motion ensures that each part of the hand is massaged and stimulated.

These simple exercises were difficult for Viva at first, not only because of her physical weakness, but because they released so much emotion. After each of our early sessions together, Viva left feeling exhausted. She had a lot of difficulty knowing how much she could do physically, and also what her limits were and when she needed to rest. So I began to teach her relaxation exercises.

I instructed her to imagine her body as very heavy, then as very light. I had her picture her blood pouring through her veins, flowing from her head down through her neck. As it reached her chest, she could feel the emotional tension slowly dissolve. She visualized blood flowing through the muscles of her back, her solar plexus, the muscles and organs of her abdominal cavity, into her pelvis, down her legs, and into her feet. She would spend at least five minutes imagining the blood circulating through her feet, imagining each toe growing warm, before visualizing the blood going back up her legs and through the rest of her body, until it reached into her hands. I asked her to feel the connection between the toes of her left foot and the fingers of her left hand. By doing so, she encouraged the neurological communication between these two areas. This feeling of inter-connectedness increases one's ability to influence the body's functioning, which in turn produces more circulation and vitality.

Gradually Viva began to overcome her fatigue. After two months of treatment, both our sessions and her exercises became a little easier for her. Still, she complained to me that she frequently felt exhausted. "Why don't you do the relaxation exercises each time you feel exhausted!" I yelled at her. And she responded, "I didn't know I was supposed to. I thought they were for the exercise period."

"Why don't you listen to your body and not just do what you think you are supposed to?" I asked. Viva was silent.

After this, whenever Viva felt fatigued, regardless of what she was doing, she did her relaxation exercises, even if briefly, and then returned to her activity refreshed. After a few more months, her fatigue disappeared and her hands and feet were warm all of the time. I knew then that she was cured from anemia, and her blood tests later confirmed this. She felt and acted as if she had come back to life. This whole process took five months.

In the final analysis, most physical problems are in some way related to poor circulation. We work on strengthening the circulation of every patient who comes to us. While good circulation alone might not bring about a cure, no cure is really possible without it.

Dvora had undergone eleven operations for a serious hernia condition. She was an Orthodox Jewish woman, which meant that her life and activities were severely limited. Having to observe the many religious strictures was a burden to her, and her slow walk and stooped posture reflected this. Her husband was a self-centered, demanding man who asked a lot more of her than he was willing to give back. He treated her more like a servant than a life companion.

Her shoulders were stiff and tense, and this tension worked its way into every muscle of her body. Though she believed devoutly in her religion, living with so many restrictions left scars of anger and resentment in both her body and her personality. She was a compassionate, generous woman, receptive to new ideas and open to other people. She took care of her family, including her mentally unstable brother, and of everyone and everything around her. She also cared for herself, which was why she came to us despite her husband's scorn.

When I first saw Dvora, it was obvious she needed to make some major changes in her life. She had lost the inner source of strength in a life of catering to the needs of others. She needed to find it and to build a life around that strength. The expression on her face when she walked into my office was something I will never forget. A compassionate and tender soul was hidden behind a tough, aggressive look which had become habitual through years of conflict. Yet her dark eyes were warm and vital.

I knew Dvora had to learn to breathe. After one hundred slow, deep breaths, she felt very relaxed and certain that she would get better, both physically and mentally. I explained to her how we would strengthen all the muscles of her abdomen, so that the muscles around her intestines would not rupture again. Her muscles were weak and degenerated, but I was sure she would make whatever effort she needed to improve. The expression in her eyes had already softened and expressed her whole loving soul. She reminded me of my grandmother, who is for me the personification of selfless love, and of Miriam, who led me to vision.

The first exercise was very important. One reason she always felt so weighted down was lack of oxygen. Her breathing was shallow and rapid. I taught her to concentrate on her breathing, first by counting the length of each exhalation and inhalation to achieve longer, deeper breaths, and then by consciously expanding her abdomen as she breathed. This helped her relax and feel lighter, and it strengthened her abdominal muscles.

I massaged her abdomen, and the muscles responded immediately. The tighter ones became looser, and the weaker, dead-feeling ones became firmer. Next, I put one hand on her abdomen and the other on her lower back, and told Dvora to visualize the two hands meeting inside her abdomen. I told her to imagine that my hands, which were opening, warming, and loosening the muscles of her abdomen and back, were doing the same to her internal muscles, relaxing the entire abdominal cavity. Then I taught her to massage her own abdomen, and while she lacked sensitivity, she was able to relax the muscles a little. She breathed more deeply, and felt great relief by the time she left.

During our next session, while massaging and relaxing Dvora, I gave her a third exercise. Normally while walking she would just drag her heavy legs, letting her abdominal and lower back muscles contract and do all the work. She had, in fact, a tendency to use her entire body to perform any motion, exerting far more effort than was necessary. This kept her body tense and weak. I asked her to consciously direct her legs to work for themselves. She of course had a deep resistance to changing her habit. Through deep breathing and constantly reminding herself to use only her legs for walking (or whatever specific muscles were needed for any particular movement), she was able to do this sometimes during our sessions and her exercise periods. My goal was for Dvora to make correct and effortless movement automatic.

Dvora's husband opposed her treatment with me and refused to support it, so she took a part-time job to cover the expense of the treatment. She told me that she thanked God that she could see me while her husband was at work to avoid arguing with him about it. Meanwhile, she was making very significant improvements. Her hernia pains would recur occasionally, but the visualization exercise in which she would imagine my hands going through her abdomen and back and meeting inside, nearly always relieved the pain. Within three months, her body became much stronger, particularly the abdominal muscles. But she still felt weighed down emotionally. Her daughter, who was nine years old and still wetting the bed, was affected by her mother's suffering and by the problems between her parents.

One day Dvora came to our center smiling and cheerful, ready to begin our work. She had done her homework, and it was clear to both of us that she had improved greatly. I asked her to breathe deeply and after a few warm-up exercises and some massage, I lifted one of her legs and asked her to feel its heaviness as I held it. I set it down and asked her to imagine I was lifting it again. Even imagining me lifting her leg made her feel how hard it was to just relax and allow it to be lifted. She grew flushed and nauseated, as if she were straining to lift the leg herself.

Then I asked her to lift the leg, and she found this easier than the visualization, as she could use her stomach muscles to assist the leg. In actually performing the motion, she reverted to her old ways, allowing other muscles to work for her legs, but in visualization she couldn't. She was so dependent on her abdomen, back and pelvis to help her move the leg, that the image of lifting it by its own power overwhelmed her. I tried once again to get her to visualize letting the leg lift itself, and once more she grew flushed and nauseated. When I asked her to imagine lifting both legs together, she actually passed out for a moment.

This experience was overwhelming for her. For the first time, Dvora fully experienced the effects of tension, and she saw clearly that her tension was caused by the way she used her body. She realized what she had to do, and she decided to do it. She left my office that day feeling heavy and a little sick, but with a deep sense of challenge and self-confidence.

Dvora was never the same. From then on, she was able to cope with all of her physical problems and she found imagery her most useful tool. She improved the way she did her exercises, and she reached the point where she could raise and lower both legs, together or separately, with little or no effort. But the most complete sense of release she felt was by visualizing herself lying on her back and lifting her feet until they stretched behind her head, and rolling forward until her hands touched her toes. She could not actually do these motions, but imagining them helped her immensely.

She began working on herself with the devotion she showed her family and the Hebrew commandments. She grew stronger and felt lighter in body and spirit, and her life changed completely. Her relationship with her husband began to improve – at least from her viewpoint – as she learned to stand up for herself. Her daughter's and brother's problems became a priority as she was now capable of handling them without harming herself.

It was wonderful to see her blossom, in the middle of her life. Her progress was extremely rapid once she realized what she had been doing wrong. By releasing destructive tensions and learning to relax, she had the energy to rebuild herself, and her muscles grew stronger all the time until she was completely cured.

Up until then, she had been offered only symptomatic treatment for a deep-rooted problem. Only her ruptured muscles had been dealt with, and not the emotional and physiological pressures which caused the damage. Doctors had been able to fuse the torn muscles surgically, but they could not prevent recurrent ruptures. Addressing only effects and not causes is at best unsatisfactory, and can actually be dangerous. When Dvora learned to heal her body at its deepest, most basic level, she not only learned to treat her hernia problem, but she gained the capacity to prevent future recurrences.

After three months of working with Naomi, the spine patient I mentioned earlier, I decided it was time for us to begin strengthening her legs, abdomen, and lower back. The first exercise I gave her was to raise both legs together while lying on her back. She could barely lift even one leg without a great deal of effort. I told her to visualize her leg as being very heavy and short – short, because muscles shorten as they contract. As she practiced this imagery and tried to lift one leg, her lower back tensed, and she felt that she could hardly breathe. Next I told her to imagine that the leg was normal in size and in weight. As she did this, her back relaxed and her breathing returned to normal. Then I told her to imagine that the leg had grown longer and was as light as a cloud. When she did this, the muscles of her back relaxed completely, lying almost flat against the table. This visualization exercise helped Naomi feel the connection between her legs and her back, and after doing it, she was able to lift her leg without tensing any other muscles. This gave her a great deal of relief. After we did this with the other leg, I asked Naomi to visualize lifting both her legs up and down twenty times. A severe pain developed in her forehead, so I massaged it to relieve the pain. Gradually she could not only visualize lifting both legs, but she was able to actually lift them successfully.

Visualization has become essential to our therapy. I have found it to be beneficial to every part of the body, and for certain individuals, it has been the key to solving their physical problems. Imagery is important because it helps us recognize our unconscious feelings and conceptions about our bodies. Sometimes change can come about through awareness alone, but it generally takes time and work. Naomi had not realized that she subconsciously believed it to be very difficult for her to raise her leg, nor that as a result of this belief, she was putting far too much effort into a simple motion. When she realized how difficult it was to even imagine lifting her leg, her whole attitude changed. She realized immediately how much her mind affected her body's movement.

Once someone recognizes her problems and their causes, it is much easier to find a solution. The therapist's main job is to help the patient increase her awareness. Visualization is a very effective tool for this. I have found it to be most effective when used in conjunction with massage and movement. If a patient has tense muscles in her leg, the therapist may hold and gently stretch it while asking the patient to imagine that the muscles are growing longer, lighter, and looser, or that the breath is flowing into the tight muscles, through the leg and out of the feet. In nearly every case, the muscles will indeed lengthen and relax.

The therapist must of course be creative. The same visualization exercise is not right for every patient and it is up to the therapist to find which imagery will help the patient. Once she learned how helpful visualization was, Naomi continued to use it along with her exercises with great success, until gradually her back became strong and healthy.

Chapter 12

Muscular dystrophy

Touch is the primary tool in the treatment of muscular dystrophy. A healing touch is the first requirement of the muscular dystrophy patient; it must do for him what he is, at first, too weak to do for himself. The touch which heals is one which is sensitive and responsive to the condition and needs of an individual patient. Physical therapy as practiced today has become too standardized and formalized a method to be able to supply to each individual what he needs. A muscular dystrophy patient needs to learn to care for his muscles, both in order to resist the process of decay, and gradually to rebuild those muscles which have become wasted. Any disease causes destruction in some part of the body, but the body is, given the right conditions, capable of overcoming the disease. With the right kind of support, whether it be rest, medication, nutrition, activity, tender loving care, or whatever the body most needs, a patient can overcome the most virulent of diseases, and can return to normal, perhaps even stronger than before the disease struck.

With muscular dystrophy patients the crucial question is: how far have the muscles already decayed when treatment is first undertaken? How much has the patient still to work with? The sooner treatment is begun, the better the chance of the patient returning to normal.

Massage increases circulation in the muscles, something

the patients themselves are unable to do through exercise. The supply of vital nutrients to the cells is thus increased. Massage aids in neuromuscular transmissions by stimulating the nerves. Respiration becomes deeper and easier as the patient being massaged begins to relax, increasing the supply of oxygen to the entire body. It has been suggested that muscles of muscular dystrophy patients become exhausted as the result of insufficient calcium absorption. Whatever the reason, it is clear that the muscles of a muscular dystrophy patient are completely lacking in energy. Massage has been demonstrated to help bring fresh energy to exhausted muscles, making more vigorous movement possible. This energy can be obtained by the muscular dystrophy patient in no other way.

It is very important that MD patients receive proper and adequate rest during the course of the treatment. Many patients do damage to themselves by trying to function normally; these efforts cause a great strain and overloading of muscles and nerves. We have found that any sort of strain placed upon the weakened tissues of a muscular dystrophy patient is destructive. These tissues must be strengthened through massage before they can be asked to perform in any capacity.

It is of the utmost importance for a therapist to be able to sense the proper amount of pressure to apply when touching his patient. This is true in treating any kind of disorder, but it is essential with muscular dystrophy cases. The treatment of muscular dystrophy requires a very light touch, and the therapist must be able to assess, not only the degree of pressure required for each patient, but the degree of pressure needed for each individual group of muscles. Tissue which has not yet deteriorated but has become strained, requires a much firmer touch than a muscle which has begun to decay. The warmth of the therapist's hands is instrumental in creating stimulation, relaxation, and a feeling of energy in the patient's muscles. Massage, if done correctly, can both relax and strengthen muscles. The therapist must be aware of the muscles' degree of weakness and fatigue, and their capacity for movement. An incorrect touch may tire, tense or even damage the muscles. A sensitive therapist can use massage as the catalyst for stimulating the body's own healing and regenerative processes to act. Choice of technique, amount of pressure applied through the fingers of the therapist, level of concentration and commitment, knowledge of when to end a session – all these aspects of sensitivity and knowledge contribute to the effectiveness of the therapy. Even the gentlest touch at the wrong time, when the patient is tired, can have disastrous effects on the muscles.

The next step in the treatment of muscular dystrophy is the use of "passive" movement; that is, movement in which parts of the patient's body are moved by the therapist rather than by the patient himself, during the course of the massage. A gentle and penetrating massage can be as vigorous and stimulating for an MD patient as running is to a normal person. It increases both the speed and the pressure of the circulation, pumping the blood into the tissues, which increases the supply of oxygen throughout the body. It helps the blood to carry away deposits of waste materials, and in general greatly enhances the condition of the muscles. Massage also increases the thickness of the tissues being massaged. Passive movement should be used only after the patient's muscles have had the benefit of the massage, and should be done carefully.

Passive movement has many benefits. It releases the tensions in those muscles which have become strained through doing the work of the weaker muscles. These over-worked muscles are almost perpetually contracted, and feel hard and tight, which indicates strain and fatigue, rather than decay. We refer to these contracted muscles as "malnourished," because in their contracted state they are restricting the flow of blood, lymph, and other vital fluids, and are unable to receive or utilize their necessary supply of nutrients and oxygen. This state of contraction is responsible for many problems which arise in the body. In an MD patient, this problem is intensified, because those muscles are working for ones which are not only habitually unused, but have actually deteriorated so that they are *incapable* of doing what is required of them. If two muscles are holding a bone in place, and one of them becomes weaker, the stronger muscle will pull the bone towards itself, out of its proper alignment. In trying to function normally, the MD patient puts enormous stress on his functioning muscles, which are under attack from the same disease which has already destroyed the non-functioning muscles. This strain and effort speeds up the disease process.

Passive movement re-accustoms the muscles to movement, without requiring them to struggle against gravity or resistance. It allows functional and non-functional muscles to enjoy the benefits of mild exercise, without tiring them. A circular, or rotating, motion is most helpful, as it includes within its scope *all* the muscles which should be used in a particular motion, rather than emphasizing only a few of them. The tendency to overwork a few muscles particularly needs to be corrected in patients who do not have the capacity for equal use of all their muscles. The movement should also be suited to the muscles involved; weak muscles must be moved gently and repeatedly, whereas strong but contracted muscles may be stretched more vigorously. In cases of muscular dystrophy, patients require hundreds of hours of massage and thousands of hours of passive movement before the muscles can be built up to where they can perform exercises by themselves actively.

This is our basic pattern of treatment for muscular dystrophy: massage, passive movement, and then active movement, gently and gradually increasing in intensity and duration. We have documented the use of this treatment in rebuilding atrophied and dystrophic muscles. Every muscular dystrophy patient treated by us has shown thickening and strengthening of muscle fibers which had originally degenerated. The rebuilding of atrophied muscles is a very difficult and demanding task. It requires the total commitment of the therapist, the patient, and the patient's family.

The Vegetarian Society hosted many conferences on health and medicine which were attended by prestigious physicians and health care professionals. It was at one of these conferences that we had met Dr Arkin, the neurologist, who also practiced acupuncture.

Even though Vered's improvement was remarkable, she still limped heavily. Vered and I told Dr Arkin what we had done for her so far, and asked him if he could do anything for her leg. He was very interested and invited us to his home to meet with him informally.

We brought Danny along as well, and Dr Arkin was most impressed at the muscle development Danny showed in his arms and his thighs. He could see at once that Danny's muscles were ones which in most people were underdeveloped, but which Danny had built up to replace ones which had deteriorated.

Dr Arkin examined my eyes and was stunned when he saw the fragmented lenses. "With these lenses you should be completely blind," he told me.

In answer to our original question, Dr Arkin told us that there was nothing that acupuncture could do to increase Vered's mobility and that our method was probably the best thing in the world for her. But he was very interested in Danny. In Danny's pilgrimage from clinic to clinic in search of a cure, he had been to Dr Arkin's clinic; and Dr Arkin thus had access to Danny's records. He was able to appreciate the enormous improvement Danny had made, and this more than anything else convinced him of the value of our work.

Danny's form of muscular dystrophy, the Duchenne type, is considered to be a genetic disease, characterized by progressive atrophy and wasting of the muscles. Onset is usually at an early age, and it occurs more frequently in males than in females. Its cause is thought to be a genetic defect in muscle metabolism. There is no known medical cure.

There are many different forms of muscular dystrophy. Some, like the Duchenne type, are very severe, usually occurring in childhood and leading rapidly to decay of the muscles, paralysis, and death. Others, like facio-scapulo-humeral muscular dystrophy, affect a more localized area of the body and produce a more gradual atrophy, leading eventually to increasing weakness and to partial or total paralysis, but are not usually fatal. The disease attacks only the striated or skeletal muscles. These are the external, fibrous muscles which are used in the performance of voluntary motion. Although researchers are not certain what causes MD, they persist in seeking a chemical cure, even though it is still not known if in fact it has a chemical cause.

In normal practice, MD patients are given no hope. They are told to expect a gradual, progressive deterioration, and eventually death. In the case of Duchenne muscular dystrophy, death usually occurs before the age of 18, and more often in early childhood. The older the child is at the onset of the disease, the longer the decay process takes, as there is more muscle tissue to be destroyed. Rarely does Duchenne MD attack someone later than puberty.

Dr Arkin referred a patient to us who had an unusual case of muscular dystrophy. Mr Kominski was 50 years old when he came to us. The process of deterioration had begun when he was twenty and developed very slowly over thirty years. Until a year earlier, he had seemed almost normal, but then his condition worsened dramatically. He owned a small citrus farm, and he began to have a difficult time picking fruit because he could barely lift his arms. He had consulted several doctors and faith healers, to no avail.

I tested his muscles and found that his pectoral muscles were very contracted and had almost completely atrophied. His throat was so tight he could hardly speak. His arm muscles too were tight and hard, and his arms could barely move. The few leg muscles he could still use were extremely tight, even when he was at rest. This indicated that they were working far beyond their capacity.

I told Mr Kominski that he had to stop pushing himself beyond his limits when his muscles were in such a state of exhaustion. Our first suggestion was that he immediately stop certain activities, particularly the hard labor of caring for his orchard and fields. He needed to become aware of his weakness and then work on strengthening himself.

I went to work massaging his muscles, which was a great relief to him, though it was several sessions before the results of the treatment showed. Gradually Mr Kominski began to feel more energetic and to function better. We grew to like each other very much. At our suggestion, he consulted Dr Frumer for a natural diet. He stopped eating meat and began a diet of simple, unprocessed foods, which helped his worn-out body by making digestion easier and lowering the level of toxic material the body had to eliminate. Mr Kominski's main problem was that he simply had no idea what was helpful for his body and what was not.

After only three weeks, he had improved so significantly – finding it much easier to use his arms, walk, and to function in general – that he went to his neurologist, Dr Kotter, to show her what had happened to him. As the chief neurologist at her hospital, she had a staff of thirteen neurologists under her. She called a meeting to show them, along with a group of medical students, the improvement in Mr Kominski's muscles. His case seemed to confirm her own ideas – that what a patient with muscular dystrophy needs most of all is the right kind of movement therapy.

Dr Kotter asked to meet us. This made me quite nervous, as I was barely twenty and completely without conventional training, so I called Dr Arkin, who reassured me that she was a very open-minded person and that I should by all means meet with her.

The first thing we did was show her the documents of Danny's medical history, and she was so impressed with his progress that she expressed doubts that he had ever had muscular dystrophy. Our visit with Dr Kotter was cordial, and for the chief neurologist of a major hospital she gave us quite a compliment in saying, "One thing I know for sure – you three are authentic. There is a lot you don't know, and I will straighten you out anytime you say something that doesn't make sense to me as a doctor. But I like what you are doing, and I will refer patients to you to see what sort of results you get." From a person in her position, this was warm praise.

A few weeks later, Dr Kotter referred Lili to us. She told Lili's father that there was nothing that could be done medically to help his daughter, who suffered from muscular dystrophy. "As for nutrition, you can feed her any soup you want, but I don't think it will help either. But I do know three young people who might be able to help her. If you see them, please tell me the results."

Lili was five years old. She had shown the first symptoms of muscular dystrophy at eighteen months and had already outlived her first doctor's prognosis. Although she could barely crawl, her parents never got her a wheelchair, suspecting that this might cause her psychological trauma. I was pleased about this, because sitting in a wheelchair would have robbed her of the little opportunity she had for movement.

Lili was very weak and her body was thin and deformed. Her hands flopped to the side and could not be held forward. Her shoulder blades and collar bone bulged out of their sockets, barely covered with skin. Her back was curved into the shape of a banana. Her neck was so weak that her head lolled forward on her chest. When she crawled, it was with an ineffective sideways groping, rather than straight forward like a normal child. She was hardly breathing.

The first time we tested her we found that it was difficult

for her to lift her arms. She could not move them at all against any resistance. Nor could she lift her legs, and when we asked her to lie on her stomach and bend her knee, she could only raise the foot a few inches. Any normal motion was next to impossible for her. She had no strength in her body. We prescribed massage and passive movement, that is, movement which is done by the therapist rather than the patient, in which part of the patient's body is held and gently moved by the therapist. This is quite different from physical therapy. In physical therapy, if you have a weak muscle, you are usually encouraged to work it strenuously. We tried to move Lili's weak muscles in the easiest way possible, and then showed her how to continue this movement on her own.

We showed her mother how to move Lili's foot in rotating motion, and then her leg, knee, elbow, and arm, and each toe and finger, while Lili lay on her back moving her head from side to side. After two sessions, Lili's mother called to tell us that Lili had remembered all the exercises. She even corrected some errors her mother made in helping her. Lili was wonderfully alert and perceptive, and after a couple of sessions, she became enthusiastic about her treatment and her exercises. I would say that she seemed to sense a great change coming and this awareness helped end her process of decay.

After three sessions, Lili suffered no further loss of function. With her mother's help, she did four hours of exercise each day. By the end of our fifth session, she could lie on her back and lift her leg until it was at right angles to her body, and she could lift her arms straight up over her head. Her neck muscles also began to gain in strength and mobility, although her head still drooped forward. After seven sessions, she could crawl on her hands and knees, like a normal child.

A few weeks after our first session, Lili took her first steps in three years. Her back was still deformed, with a pronounced swayback, which made it difficult for her to stand up, so I had to support her back to help her stand. I was supporting her back with one hand and her abdomen with the other, and she took a few steps!

Less than a week later, Lili was able, with some support, to walk down the stairs to her mother's car. This was the most rapid, dramatic progress I have ever seen with a muscular dystrophy patient. The joy of seeing this little girl on her feet was so powerful it has never left me. She was one of our most astonishing cases. It took only 21 days for her transformation from near-paralysis to walking.

Needless to say, our work with Lili won us the respect of Dr Kotter, who began to refer many more patients to us. It was a pleasure to work in harmony with the established medical community. We wanted to reach as many people as possible, and the support of physicians was very helpful.

Six years ago, a woman from Kodiak, Alaska, came to San Francisco to work with me on her eyes. Since she could not stay and wanted to continue working with me, she organized a workshop in Kodiak. Kodiak is an island in the Aleutian chain, the second-largest island in the United States. It is kept relatively warm by ocean currents from Japan and is full of spectacular scenery. I was warmly welcomed by the villagers, most of whom are fishing people.

The workshop was a three-day overview of everything I had learned to date. It was a memorable experience for me and, I believe, for all the participants. The concentration of the work and the large group created an intensity which helped me guide many people through physical, emotional, and even spiritual growth.

At the beginning of the workshop, I asked people to introduce themselves. That was when I met Steve. He was hunched over, unkempt, and forlorn-looking. Even through his down vest, I could see that his shoulders were emaciated. "I have facio-scapulo-humeral muscular dystrophy. It is hereditary; my brother Jim has it too. Is there anything I can do for it?" he asked by way of introduction.

During the workshop I had the chance to look at Steve's shoulders. The muscles of his chest, shoulders, and upper arms were terribly wasted. He could not lift his arms more than halfway up, and when he moved them they made a loud, creaking noise, not the usual cracking sound of tense necks and shoulders, but an actual creaking of the scapular and clavical bones grinding against one another. The weak, thin muscles could not hold them apart. Steve also had severe tension in his lower back, his arms, and his neck, where the muscles had grown very thick to compensate for his weak shoulders.

After the workshop, Steve came to see me for a treatment. I massaged his back and shoulders, and after only that much he was able to lift his arms without the creaking sound. His wife, Elaine, was there to observe. She was skeptical at first, being a conventional psychologist and the daughter of a physician. But even she could see that as I massaged the muscles of his chest, they appeared to grow more substantial. As I pressed and squeezed his lower back, I released the tension there so that more blood circulated to his shoulders; and then when I massaged around his collar bone, the trapezius muscles also appeared thicker. Afterwards Steve could lift his arms nine inches higher than before.

Elaine was so completely won over that she and Steve arranged my next workshop in Kodiak. After I left, they carefully followed my instructions. Steve had been engaged in hard physical labor as a handyman, which was a strain on his shoulders, and at my suggestion he quit, and got a less strenuous job. Elaine spent an hour a day massaging Steve and helping him with his exercises. Her love and devotion made her a very effective therapist. Steve worked on himself four hours each day, doing head and neck rotations, bending exercises, leg stretches, and gentle movements of his shoulders, wrists, elbows, and hands to loosen his overworked muscles and to build up his dystrophic muscles.

I saw Steve a year later. He could rotate his shoulders,

open and close his hands, move his forearms, hands, and elbows in rotating motion with no strain, and lift his arms and move them completely normally with no creaking. His chest and shoulder muscles were noticeably thicker. Steve's disposition had also improved. He had been irritable, angry, and impatient. These are all emotions which are used to cover a sense of weakness, frustration, and powerlessness. With his new strength came new confidence and emotional stability. He and Elaine lived simply, in a forest cabin in one of the most beautiful places in the world. Yet even this tranquil, unpressured environment had not been enough to give Steve peace of mind. Only the gentle, gradual strengthening of his body had accomplished that. The work on his body had been a labor of love, both from himself and from his wife, and it had physically and spiritually uplifted him.

During the years since then, Steve has continued to build up his muscles, and they now appear completely normal. His goal accomplished, Steve realizes that he will never be "finished" working on his body. His disease provided him with a vehicle for improving every aspect of his life and becoming more alive.

Chapter 13

Eye problems

During our time at the Vegetarian Society, when our practice was flourishing, a successful eye patient of mine asked me if I would see her son, who was the head opthalmologist in Dr Kotter's hospital. I was hesitant to see a man whose ideas about treating the eyes were bound to be opposed to my own, but his mother assured me that he was an open-minded person. I later found out she had coaxed him into meeting me in the same way.

The morning before meeting Dr Zimmerman, I spent a long time on my eye exercises. Relaxed and confident about my work, I let his mother take me to his office at the hospital. Dr Zimmerman turned out to be a pleasant young man with a beautiful broad grin. He listened with great interest to my story and my theories. When he looked at my eyes, he said he would have done a better job with the surgery, and he told me that my lenses looked like glass which had been dropped and stepped on. Then he tested my vision and simply could not believe how much I was able to see, or that it was possible for my eyes to accommodate light at all.

We disagreed about many things. He could not believe that glasses are harmful. I explained to him Dr Bates' idea that glasses weaken the eyes by preventing them from working for themselves and by focusing more light on to the macula (the center of the retina which sees detail best) than the macula can comfortably accept. He did, however, believe that eye exercises can be effective for some problems. But he could not accept the idea that the shape of the eye could actually change.

After our conversation, which was polite and stimulating for both of us, he expressed no great interest in pursuing my methods himself, so we parted as if this conversation were complete and we wouldn't need to see one another again. His mother, undaunted, decided that if her son would not pursue this with me, she would find another doctor who would and she talked a colleague of Dr Zimmerman's into trying my work.

Dr Shem had eye problems himself, and he met me at Mrs Zimmerman's home. "You can't do anything unconventional at the hospital," she told me. I taught him relaxation exercises and sunning, and by the end of the session, he was so relaxed he fell asleep. Exercising the eyes was totally new to him.

After the session, Dr Shem practiced his eye exercises faithfully, and experienced some improvement in his vision. This delighted him, not only because of the improvement, but because he felt so bold and adventurous. He continued to exercise for several months, and improved his vision considerably.

I met one other ophthalmologist at Mrs Zimmerman's home, who told me flatly that eye exercises have no value at all, that it was a myth. He said it was impossible to measure any objective results from eye exercises. I found this amusing, since the "objective" findings of ophthalmological testing vary from day to day, even hour to hour, if these tests are repeated. Eye doctors overlook the constant changes in visual acuity which every individual experiences, because they see patients for only a few minutes, and base their knowledge on what they find in those few minutes. Everyone knows that eyes see worse when they are tired, overworked, or in distress. Why this is not generally understood among ophthalmologists is a mystery to me.

Ophthalmology has many sophisticated tools to use in its fight against eye disorders, but in my opinion it remains primitive. There is no science of preventive ophthalmology. Perhaps it will be necessary to find cures for all the "critical" eye problems before the idea of preventive ophthalmology can be taken seriously. I am sure that Dr Bates' clear, straightforward theories will some day be endorsed by conventional eye doctors and not just by the patients who have benefited from them.

The Bates method is very effective and based on sound and workable ideas. Bates had an approach which genuinely helped people to cure their eye problems, and not just common eye problems but some very serious, degenerative eye diseases. He did not consider his findings to be in opposition to the spirit of his profession, but rather a means of widening the horizons of ophthalmology. However, no profession has ever welcomed sweeping changes in its practices. Bates was not only discredited, but lost his license to practice. Though his ideas were rejected by conventional ophthalmology, he continued to help thousands of people to overcome their eye problems. Pioneers in any field are often persecuted and forced to fight for what they consider worthwhile and true.

Bates always stressed that his method is in fact not a fixed method, but must be adjusted subtly to meet each individual's particular needs. While describing his exercises, he also said that if a patient is not helped by the exercises in Bates' book, that person should try to develop new exercises by experimenting as Bates himself had done. Bates understood that there is no one technique that will help everyone. Relaxation is the only consistently effective factor.

Bates understood that eye problems can result from worry and stress, as well as from an unhealthy environment. Environmental factors which may be harmful to vision include poor light, noise, air pollution, and the lack of distant horizons which give the eyes a chance to "stretch."

Boredom is another factor. When we are bored, there is a tendency to stop focusing and let the eyes "glaze over." This habit, which may lead to myopia and astigmatism, often begins in childhood. The typical classroom is a very unhealthy atmosphere for the eyes. Children spend six hours a day in an enclosed space, artificially lit, trying to pay attention to lessons which are too frequently boring or frustrating. They begin to stare vacantly or let their eyes wander aimlessly, which blurs the vision and may cause permanent damage. It is no wonder that so many children who enter school with perfectly healthy eyes need glasses by the time they are nine years old. No damage to the eyes, however, need be irreversible. By recognizing the causes of bad vision and creating healthy conditions for the eyes, all the harm that has been done may be undone.

At the age of eighty, my Aunt Esther had an auto accident and broke her leg. She was bedridden for three months while the leg was healing, and at the end of that time, a neurologist told her she had Parkinson's disease. He recommended that she have physical therapy to prevent her joints from stiffening and degenerating.

Aunt Esther phoned me and asked if I would be her therapist. My schedule at that time was completely full, so I gave up my morning exercises at the beach to work on her. I enjoyed those sessions at the beach immensely, and I knew Aunt Esther would be a difficult patient, but I really couldn't turn her down. As it turned out, she was completely uncooperative. She would not work on herself outside of our sessions. She accepted the treatments as her due and was not interested in how she might enhance them.

When I first came to see her, she was not able to get out of bed. After a month of loosening her joints, and reducing her tremors through relaxation exercises and meditation, we began to walk together, and I showed her how to walk properly. One time we walked to a lovely wooded area with a small stream near her house. As we sat down on a bench, Aunt Esther asked me, "How is it you know so much?" It was as if she knew nothing about the years I had been working on myself and on others. Only after she felt the effects of my work herself did it occur to her that my endeavors might have some validity. It impressed her that this treatment had gotten her out of bed in just one month.

I told her about Miriam, Isaac, Shlomo, and the many other people I had worked with. This seemed to make sense to her, though she said, "You still should get a degree in physical therapy." When she suggested this several years earlier, it was her way of denigrating my work, but this time she said it respectfully to encourage my obtaining credentials so that this work might be accepted more widely.

Aunt Esther's illness brought us closer. We both enjoyed the time we spent together. She felt less need to control me, and she indicated more and more that I was doing the right thing. She was particularly impressed when she learned that a half-million people had listened to my interview on the radio. At the end of her treatment, Aunt Esther presented me with a wonderful gift – a plane ticket to America.

I knew that I had the best chance of earning official credentials in America. And I realized that going to America would offer me a chance of exposure to a much greater number of people. I had begun to feel that my practice had gone as far as it could in Israel. Our center was nationally known, thanks to the radio show and extensive word-of-mouth publicity. Despite very long hours of work, Danny, Vered, and I could not see all the people who wanted to see us. It occurred to me that becoming better known and accredited would attract more practitioners, which would make our therapy available to more people. I wanted eventually to set up a hospital where our methods could be used.

My sister Bella had been living in San Francisco for some time, and she suggested that I join her there while pursuing a graduate degree in physical therapy. I had already been rejected by two conventional schools of physical therapy, and I feared that even in America my methods would be opposed. So I compromised and decided to go to San Francisco for two years to complete my undergraduate education and then return to Israel.

Bella met me at the airport and took me home. I could barely believe it was real. I felt as if I embodied the thousands of miles I had just travelled from Israel to America. As I fell asleep on Bella's couch, I felt as though I was still up in the air.

It took about a week for me to realize that this really was a totally different place. The most striking difference was that I had no patients. I had the strongest urge to work – not to be able to work was the worst fate I could imagine. It was incredibly quiet. At home in Israel the phone rang every five minutes and I would meet friends everywhere. I felt as though I were wasting time when there was so much to be done.

I had had so much support from physicians in Israel that I decided to contact doctors in California to see if one might help me get started working here. I had absolutely no success. Some were polite but couldn't imagine how to help me, and most dismissed me without a word.

Finally after six months, I received a letter from Israel with the phone number of an Alexander teacher in California. We arranged to meet, and he told me he would do his best to refer patients to me. He also introduced me to an optometrist he knew named Dr Gottlieb.

Dr Gottlieb was the first person in America who seemed to completely understand and appreciate what I had to say. He had an excellent practice, but he felt dissatisfied with it. "I myself did Bates exercises," he said. "I had a slight case of myopia, and I improved it within a year and a half. Now my vision is normal or better. But I feel the real experience of it evaded me, even though I worked hard and improved

169

my vision." I knew what he meant. "Maybe you worked too hard at the exercises instead of just experiencing them," I suggested.

I gave Dr Gottlieb a few treatments. His abdomen was very tight, and I helped him release the tension by contracting and then relaxing every muscle there, and by massaging and stretching each of his limbs. I stretched his arm while he visualized the arm reaching across the room, across the street, across the ocean, which relaxed his shoulders and chest. Afterwards, he stood more solidly on the ground, and even his face was more relaxed.

With his initial approval of my work confirmed, I began to go to his office one day a week to work with a few patients. The people I saw turned out to be quite interested in the work and the exercises, but most of them were not at all diligent about practicing between sessions. They were very open to new ideas but they really did nothing substantial with them.

I began to notice how little self-confidence the people I met in California have. In Israel it is quite different. I knew that with confidence in what you are doing, you can put your full effort behind it, and improve your vision and your health. I didn't know how to work with Americans, whose lack of self-confidence surprised me. Coming from a country constantly under the threat of war, I thought that Americans, whose country is stable and powerful, should have nothing to fear. But I soon learned that everyone feels there is something that he may lose and much that he must protect. Not even sure what it is they are protecting, people take a stance of general defensiveness. This attitude of self-protection was evident in the posture of many people I met here. As I began to better understand these new people I was working with, my work and results improved.

Dr Gottlieb and I opened a treatment center together in San Francisco. He encouraged me to teach vision improvement classes. Until then I had only worked with individuals, and

I was not sure my work would be effective with groups of people. I soon found out that in a small class which met for three or four hours, I could establish an atmosphere of closeness and give each student enough individual attention. Everyone who stayed with the course improved his or her vision, but some people found ingenious ways to avoid plunging into something unfamiliar. My technique demanded that the students change their whole way of seeing, and some people responded by calling the work difficult or time-consuming, and leaving the course mid-way through. Over the years fewer and fewer students leave my classes early, but I think I was a little too brash and direct during these first years in America.

Still, I found that I could teach students how to develop kinesthetic awareness and also the basic principles behind my work. On the whole, the classes were a success. Dozens of students completed them and improved their vision. I am very grateful to Dr Gottlieb for helping me get started in America. After a year together, we had learned what we were able to learn from one another, and we went our separate ways.

As time went on, working with individual patients became my main activity again. I didn't need to lecture or explain so much. My touch offered patients relief and strength, and they usually did not concern themselves with the theory behind it. Still, the experience of teaching was valuable for me. I did learn how to talk about my work in a way which inspired people to appreciate the importance of caring for their eyes and their bodies. I have continued to teach since then with an excellent rate of success. In my classes, students are required to work hard and really achieve some results. It is pointless to just "attend" my classes. Self-healing demands a decision to look closely at yourself and make whatever changes are necessary.

Leulia was my first major success in America. She was an

older woman who was born with double vision and crossed eyes, and she often complained of a stiff neck and back. She had been going to a chiropractor, sometimes twice a day, as well as a homeopath and an ophthalmologist. Besides her chronic problems, she had periodic eye infections. Luelia was hypersensitive to light, and she worried incessantly about her health. Whenever she came to see me, she always had a list of a dozen health problems. Despite her complaining and feelings of loneliness, she had a lot of courage and many interests. She was the editor of a small publishing company specializing in religious books. She was a very religious person, and in this she found her faith, strength, and comfort. She believed her coming to see me was divinely ordained.

Luelia was seventy years old and although she had adjusted to seeing double, her eyes were in constant pain from tension and could not be relieved by drugs. Leulia had even worked with Bates teachers, but her work had been unsuccessful. She finally gave up on both conventional and wholistic methods and decided "to put her problems in God's hands."

Luelia was visiting a museum outside Los Angeles and met a woman there who asked her if there was something wrong with her eyes. When Leulia told her her story, the woman said, "The best Bates teacher in the country lives in San Francisco," and she gave Leulia my address, which was three blocks from where Luelia lived. She was sure that God had provided an answer.

She called me the next day from Los Angeles, and on the following Sunday, instead of going to church, she came to see me. A small, frail figure with snow-white hair, Luelia had been taught by a so-called Bates teacher thirty years earlier to suppress her stronger eye and use only the weaker one. His intention had been to strengthen the weak eye, but by making it function for both eyes she had put an intolerable strain on it, and in the process weakened her good eye by under-using it. In double vision, each eye sees a separate image, and does not fuse the two into one. To tell her to suppress one eye was completely wrong. Luelia needed to learn to use both.

Another Bates teacher later insisted that she try to see a tiny dot on a page, and yelled at her when she couldn't see it, but gave her no further instruction. Many people who teach the Bates method have confused and distorted ideas about his work. When Dr Bates said that it is necessary to see even the smallest details with clarity, he did not mean that we should strain and force ourselves to do this. He meant that we should be able to learn to use our eyes in such a way that this would become possible! For Luelia it was especially wrong to strain her eyes to see.

On top of her serious physical problems, Luelia was nearly paralyzed with anxiety. She could never relax. Luelia was not able to do palming because leaning her elbows on the table made her fear she would injure her shoulders. I didn't insist that she palm, but instead I told her to sit in a very dark room, close her eyes, and imagine she saw blackness.

I understood that Luelia needed to be exposed to the self-healing method gradually, not abruptly. Patience and understanding by the therapist are often the key to a patient's success. It was important to allow her to decide what was right or wrong for her, even when I disagreed. It was important that I not impose a discipline but gradually introduce Luelia to this work and let her proceed at her own pace.

I suggested to Luelia that she allow her double vision to return, and then alternate using each eye. If it was necessary to use one eye more, it should be the stronger one. Soon she was able to read and type for more than an hour without becoming tired. Within a month of working this way, the ruptured blood vessels in her weaker eye began to heal. The whites of both her eyes cleared up and the irises became crystal clear. Whenever she was tired she sat in a dark room and tried to see black. This relaxed her and relieved any pain. Her tolerance to light increased, and she squinted less. Soon Luelia was no longer afraid of palming.

After a few months, her initial purpose in coming to me had already been accomplished. She no longer had incessant pain, and she could type for hours. But I wanted her to change not only her symptoms, but her fundamental problem as well: over-riding tension, caused by fear. Her tension was so bad that several times when she was riding in a car that passed over a small bump, she dislocated a vertebra and pinched a nerve. Her body was so tense that anything could harm her, and she was terrified of this. I needed to help her strengthen and relax her body so she would be less susceptible to her fear.

Luelia suffered from insomnia. She never slept more than two hours at a time. She told me that no one could massage her without making her scream with pain. Her body was very fragile, with many ruptured blood vessels and weak muscles. I massaged her so gently that at first it was hard for her to feel anything; she was not even aware that she was numb. As time passed, she began to participate more, both mentally and physically, in her healing. Her tension slowly lessened, and her tissues began to regain sensation. It is essential for everyone to exercise so that tension which accumulates in the muscles can be released. This was of course especially true for Luelia.

I taught her gentle and simple movements for her muscles, and after a while she could do forty minutes each day. She said this was the first time in her life that she ever did any exercises consistently. "Exercises usually just tire me out. But yours are different – they really help me." Whenever she began to get a headache, she would move her head in a rotating motion gently. She learned to massage herself, and she learned to release her lower back tension with gentle leg exercises and deep, relaxed breathing. For the first time, Luelia felt that she was in charge of her own health. In fact, she developed such confidence that during my sessions with her she began to tell me what to do.

Luelia became considerably less susceptible to pinched

nerves or a stiff neck, and her eyes improved remarkably. We dedicated one session every two weeks to her eyes. Sitting at the large window of my office, Luelia would look across the street at a shop sign. At first she saw the letters double, but overlapping. I asked her to close her eyes and imagine that there was no distance between the sign and her. She was to block out all other details and focus her attention. Then I asked her to open one eye, look at the sign, close it, and then do the same thing with the other eye. As she looked, she shifted her focus from point to point, and after a while she became able to distinguish the center of her visual field from its periphery. Although the image was still not clear, using the peripheral cells relaxed her eyes, and she could distinguish a letter or two and see the spaces between the letters. When Luelia opened both her eyes together, she saw everything distinctly double. This showed that she was beginning to correct the habit of suppressing one eye, and it was a relief for both eyes.

I had her open one eye at a time, look at the sign, then close the eye and imagine the sign as having very black letters on a very white background. She did this, first alternating eyes, and then finally with both eyes together. Soon she was able to see the whole sign clearly with each eye individually. Then I told her to close both eyes and imagine that she saw the sign first with one eye and then with the other eye, and then to imagine that she saw the sign from an angle with each eye separately. Finally, I asked her to imagine fusing these two pictures into one. When she opened her eyes, Luelia for some moments could see one crystal clear, perfectly legible image of the sign. She was utterly amazed; and from that time on her vision improved.

As her eyes relaxed more, they ceased to be crossed. This indicated that her cross-eyedness had come from tension. Sunning and palming, mental visualization exercises, and learning to look at things without effort combined to correct her vision. The idea that seeing required effort had become ingrained in her. To break this habit of straining while looking, I taught Luelia blinking exercises. Straining to see inhibits a person from blinking enough, and not blinking leads to further strain. If you try to look at a point without blinking, even for a minute, you will see how much effort this requires. Blinking rests the eyes and is essential for good vision.

I also asked Luelia to take a pen and move her eyes up and down along it as she drew a line. If she had looked at the line, she would have made an effort to see that the line was drawn straight. Seeing the line only peripherally, she could draw it without tension and consequently straighter. She repeated this exercise daily, and it helped her learn to relax while seeing with her central vision because she had become familiar with relaxing while using peripheral vision.

Luelia eventually stopped using her glasses altogether. She was permitted to drive without glasses and stopped getting eye infections. Her double vision from birth permanently disappeared at age seventy-two. You cannot help the body without helping the eyes, and vice versa. Luelia is a superb example of this.

Glasses are no cure for poor vision and offer no relief for weak eyes. They are a crutch which enables the eyes to force themselves to see; reading all the time with glasses is like walking all the time with crutches. Current ophthalmological theory contends that eyes cannot improve or change, even with exercise. This is easily disproven. Eyes do change, they change constantly, and they can always change for the better.

Part III

Vision

Chapter 14

The mind

The mind is a non-material awareness which inhabits every part of the body. Every part of the human body is a reflection of the mind. For any change to take place in the body, it must first be accepted by the mind. It is not possible to heal the body without engaging the mind's support. Unfortunately, the mind's tendency is to repeat already familiar patterns and not experiment with new ideas. This "rigidity" is manifested throughout the body.

In order to change the way we function, we must understand the premise that allows our bodies to function incorrectly in the first place: that incorrect functioning, or illness, is natural. As we are now, we cannot even imagine the possibility of perfect health. In order to attain better health, we must envision the desired improvement and practice the appropriate movement or exercise which instructs the body in the way to do it. We must work simultaneously with the mind and the body. Most health care professionals work almost entirely with the body, overlooking the fundamental importance of the mind-body connection.

The brain (as distinct from the mind) is the center of all the body's functioning. It is the mind which controls how the brain receives and reacts to the information transmitted to it by the senses. The mind establishes the patterns of perception. If I think I cannot perform some task, my mind will inform my brain that this is the case, and my brain will instruct my muscles that they cannot do it. The mind directs the senses towards which objects it should perceive, and then, through the brain, directs the functioning of the body as well. When we see, hear, taste, smell, or touch, it is the mind which determines how we experience the object.

Our minds limit our ability to utilize our brains. The brain accepts and becomes programmed for the limitations placed upon it by the mind. The entire body, including the brain, is a manifestation of a person's ideas about himself, which is to say a creation of the mind. Muscle activity is pre-patterned, always performed according to a set of rigid instructions. The muscles are simply carrying out the mind's concept of what they can do.

The mind is affected by circumstances, especially ones which affect the emotions. If you live near a highway and listen to traffic noise hour after hour, you cannot help but become irritable and tense your muscles. Frustrating or difficult life situations can make us feel tense, weak, and vulnerable, and so our bodies become tense, weak, and vulnerable.

The body's innate intelligence is prevented from expression by the limitations placed on it by the mind. This is not just a modern dilemma; it has been true for thousands of years. Instead of instinctively using the correct muscle to perform appropriately, we use whole groups of other muscles unnecessarily and inefficiently, leaving us strained and exhausted. The mind perceives this incorrect movement as normal and rigidly refuses to allow any new understanding.

No pathology or disease can occur without the full cooperation of the mind. By imposing its rigidity, via the nerves, upon the muscles, it hampers all functioning within the body. Circulation, with its vital distribution of oxygen and nutrients and equally vital cleansing action, is restricted nerve function is distorted and respiration is limited. Incalculable damage is done by prolonged muscular tension.

Pathology is inevitable when normal body functioning is disrupted. In the case of multiple sclerosis, for example, it is of little use to try to find a chemical to rebuild the myelin sheath when the patient's body, through its daily activities, is actively and continually engaged in destroying it. Multiple sclerosis and arthritis are degenerative *processes*, not diseases. Unless the cooperation of the mind is sought in reducing the tension in the body and lessening the overload on the nervous system, the nerves of the multiple sclerosis patient will continue to deteriorate.

Modern medicine is very successful at finding cures for diseases. But the pathologies which arise from the mind's rigidity, if suppressed in one form, will find another. Without addressing the fundamental problem, we will never rid humanity of disease by finding cures for particular diseases. As long as we fear disease, it will never disappear. I believe that even if we stop vaccinating children against polio, an epidemic would be unlikely to recur – the fear of the threat of polio has gone. It has been transferred to other diseases. It is useless to overcome the fear of a particular disease. It is the fear itself which we must eradicate.

Understanding that the mind governs the body is the first vital step towards understanding the body and its functions. The mind uses the body to translate thought into physical reality. A sense of oneself as being small can, through physical tension, transform even a tall person into a stooped, slumped, cramped, "small" person. Likewise a sense of strength and power can cause a small person to move with such energy and expansiveness that his or her size becomes irrelevant and may even be unnoticed. The mind can re-educate the muscles in ways that are harmful or helpful. Through the mind, the process of physical degeneration can be reversed. We can eliminate the idea of the inevitability of disease. If we feel weak, small, or helpless, we can practice exercises – physical and mental – which give us a sense of expansiveness. If we notice any tendency in the body to improve, any sign that a process of degeneration is reversing, we should do everything in our power to encourage it. We can allow the body to become more at ease with itself, more flexible, and less stressed. Even if we have undergone damage to nerves or muscles, that tissue can be regenerated through a program of mental and physical exercises. To do this we have to work with both body and mind, so that the non-material concept of health is manifested in our material being. This takes a lot of work. The loving hands of a friend, therapist, parent, or mate can help bring healthy stimulation to our muscles and nerves.

Just as the mind is the basis of everything in the physical body, the "world mind" is the source of everything in the world – all thought, actions, ideas, and feelings. It is a consciousness which is shared by all humanity. It is not infinite. It has the same limitations and patterns which humanity at any given moment imposes on itself.

Every individual is in a dialogue with the world mind. As a result, any change to any society, or any individual, affects us all. Nothing happens anywhere which is not both reflected from the world mind and back to it. The thoughts, feelings, actions, or conditions of any individual, society, or humanity itself, spring from the world mind, and by their existence perpetuate the world mind.

The similarities, assumptions, customs, and personality traits of a specific culture are a reflection in miniature of how the world mind works. Just as people develop similarly within a culture, humanity continually evolves in oneness through the world mind.

Any individual act reverberates through the world mind for all of humanity. No individual can remain unaffected by any human act, although the effects may not be experienced consciously or immediately. Every thought and act contributes to the total picture of humanity, and becomes part of the world mind.

Like the mind of an individual, the world mind tends to resist change and preserve concepts and situations which are already known. New and creative ideas come only from beyond the world mind and are rare because the world mind is so powerful.

Creating change in the world mind is the most difficult thing a person can hope to do. An individual's mind by itself presents a tremendous challenge. The idea of restored health is almost inconceivable to the muscular dystrophy patient who sees his body wasting away. It is nearly impossible for such a person to accept the idea that these muscles could be rebuilt and their strength restored. Only by demonstrating that this can be done and how it can be done can we change the world.

Our individual mind is like a clerk who prefers repetition of routine tasks to creative change, and the world mind, or mind of all humanity, is like a clerks' convention. It too often prefers repetition to creativity. But there are moments of grace or liberation when we step outside the world mind, and are momentarily free from our patterns. It is during these times that both the individual and the world mind can change.

Chapter 15

Vision: a self-healing community

A new type of hospital is needed, where therapists and patients can work together to create health. The therapists will not *cure* the patients, they will simply guide them on the path of *self*-healing. It will be up to the patients to do the work to improve their lives and their health.

Hospitals today, and in the past also, foster a dependent relationship between patients and doctors. In such an atmosphere, patients are discouraged from fully participating in their own treatment. There is no place where patients can work together with therapists to make changes necessary to become well and prevent their disease from recurring.

In the community I envision, the therapist will guide the patients and also work on themselves. They will instruct and support the patients in their therapy, and they will also provide living examples by spending a portion of each day working on themselves.

People will come here to deeply experience themselves, their sicknesses, and their health, in a way which is nearly impossible under ordinary circumstances. The transformation from habitual patterns and conventional understandings to accurate, penetrating insight takes time, and is most likely to succeed in a calm, nurturing environment. To contemplate health after years of self-destructive tendencies, we need healthful, pleasant surroundings, where we can lay aside the stresses of everyday life for a time and devote our full attention to self-healing.

For this I envision an isolated rural area, perhaps one mile square, with several central buildings and about one hundred cabins. The main hall can be used for dining and group events; the classroom building for clients and therapists to work together, individually and in small groups; and the "hospital" for therapists to observe, instruct, work with and evaluate their client's progress. The cabins should be separated by wooded areas, and connected by paths. There should be a creek and several natural pools for swimming, and a large garden, where vegetables, herbs, and flowers are organically grown, will provide a place where patients and therapists can work, if they wish.

At this community, the clients will meet frequently with each other in groups, including groups of people with the same illnesses. What could be more encouraging to a group of progressive muscular dystrophy patients than to see other MD patients building up their muscles one by one? Group meetings will provide clients with support, shared knowledge, and encouragement. Each client will have the opportunity to describe his feelings and experiences, and this is extremely beneficial. A whole group working together towards recovery has enormous power. People who think they are sicker than anyone else has ever been will see some in even worse shape and will also see others who started out worse and are now better.

Groups can exercise together and receive instruction suited to their common needs. When a group of asthma patients breathes together deeply and smoothly, they will help each other develop the strength to withstand attacks. Patients with similar problems can work on each other in groups of two to four.

Clients will work on themselves in their cabins for six to

eight hours each day. Once a week there will be a workshop led by a patient in which the entire community, including the therapists, will participate as students. Once a month, a senior therapist will lead a three-to five-day workshop for everyone. Each person will always have the option of doing something different if they prefer; even though it will be a communal situation, people can always opt for privacy if they wish.

Inner peace and the knowledge that no sickness of body or mind is inevitable will be the underlying group consciousness. Everyone will meditate on the concept of "no disease." The progress of the clients will be thoroughly documented, and if possible their treatment will be supervised by physicians.

This will not be a place of retreat, merely to escape from everyday life. Patients or therapists seeking escape from the pressures and problems of their lives are seldom open to learning or growing. They prefer to cling to familiar, rigid patterns of behavior.

I suspect very few people will actually want to come to a community like this and only a fraction will be able to stay for long. A commitment of six months will be necessary to allow enough time for the self-healing process to unfold. Our resistance to change, even to improvement, is very strong. Less than six months will not be enough time for most participants. The individuals who come at first will pave the way for many more to follow, by demonstrating the efficacy of this work, and supporting and strengthening one another.

The first step toward making the world a better place to live must be to improve the health of everyone. The only way to rid humanity of disease is for each person to become healthy, to become his or her own healer. Freed from preoccupation with painful or ailing bodies, we can concentrate our attention on deepening our awareness. From the base of individuals learning to care for their health, we can create a new world. We need to free the mind so that it will not inhibit the body from realizing its true potential.

In my workshops, I give people many different kinds of exercises. I teach them to move all parts of their bodies. If we are not moving any one portion, the rest of the body is affected. For example, paralyzed legs affect the arms and the torso. As a patient learns more movement in the rigid area of the body, he finds that normal movements in other areas become easier too. To allow more movement, he must break the patterns that perpetuate stiffness. The purpose of a community for self-healing is the same. For human beings to advance to our full potential, we have to have more movement. People who are unwell have a deep melancholy with regard to their bodies. By shaking loose that rigid connection, we will create the physical freedom necessary for perfect health and true spiritual freedom.

A revolution has been slowly and quietly taking place in the attitudes of many people towards disease and health. More and more people are realizing that it is possible to create health and not just combat sickness. Our community will reflect and lead this new awareness. Instead of perpetuating the notion that disease is normal, we will help create a world which affirms perfect health.

When I was in my twenties and already well-established in the United States, I decided to undertake an eight-day juice fast to cleanse my body. I had done this before and found it very helpful to my eyes. One of my patients drove me to the Sierra Nevada mountains to a remote area near Donner Pass. As we drove through the pass, I had sober thoughts about its history. It seemed ironic that I was coming to fast in the place where those unfortunate pioneers had starved to death.

It occurred to me that I knew people who had fasted for as long as ninety days for health reasons without endangering themselves, whereas others have starved to death in as little as three weeks. It seemed to me that the mind and the will are what make the difference. Fasting for a purpose, with determination and intention, is not like being deprived of food against your will. Fear, misery, and despair are the real problems, not deprivation of food alone. Fasting is cleansing, purifying, and restful.

I brought my juicer with me, and made vegetable and fruit juices, walked the mountain trails, and worked on myself. In my room I did deep breathing exercises and palming. In palming I enjoyed a sense of perfect relaxation and contentment. I found I was able to live comfortably on one glass of juice a day, even though I love food and generally eat a lot.

By the fourth day I was in a meditative state almost constantly. I sat down to palm and found that I could see perfect blackness, a rare achievement which means that the eyes and the optic nerve are completely at rest. The blackness deepened as I continued, and a great sense of calm spread throughout my body.

Then my eyes started to feel a sharp pain, the pain of having been overworked and strained. It disappeared after a few minutes, but then I felt pressure on my eyes, and I had a sudden, vivid memory. I recalled the time six months before when I had become so discouraged that I actually wanted to be blind again. I had been studying anatomy and physiology in college and found my reading unbearably slow, difficult, and painful. I studied day and night and still did poorly on my exams. It was just too much effort. If this was what the world of sight had to offer, forget it! I was ready to sacrifice years of work on my eyes for the simple peace of blindness.

The desire to be blind again grew so strong that I consulted a Gestalt therapist, who was able to help me. He asked me to picture a place I wanted to be, and I began by describing a room which was completely dark and very restful for my eyes. I went on to describe a brilliantly sunny garden which surrounded the room – its deep green, tropical plants; sparkling azure pools; clear, blue skies; and penetrating, golden light. The therapist smiled. "You see? You probably want to see more than anyone else in the world." As if by magic, my resistance to sight disappeared, and I wanted to see more than ever before.

The sense of pressure in my eyes that came over me during palming felt exactly like the pressure I felt during those exams, and it took nearly an hour of palming to work through it. This was followed by a terrible fatigue, and then a burning sensation. I became accustomed to these sensations during my years of studying and reading without glasses.

I then started to experience all the sensations I had ever felt in my eyes, as though I were traveling backwards in time. I felt as I had at eighteen, when I first fully experienced light in my eyes. Sometimes the light would hurt, and sometimes it would be as delicious as a warm bath. I sensed my eyes at seventeen, when the blur that I knew as vision had just begun to rearrange itself, and recognizable images would sometimes, amazingly, appear.

I went back further, to age fifteen, when I saw nothing but an empty blur, and my eyes were totally without sensation. Not only did my eyes lack sensation, my whole body had an insubstantial, unreal feeling, as though I simply did not exist. I remained here in a place of not-being for an hour, and I started to become bored. The pop music I could hear in the next room seemed more interesting than what I was doing.

Just as I was beginning to drift off, I saw the image of a baby. The baby was hardly breathing. He seemed to be suffocating, and I asked him, "Why don't you breathe?" He answered in Russian, my first language, "Because I am afraid." "What are you afraid of?" he answered. "I am afraid no one else will see what I see."

I knew that the baby was myself. I could see that his eyes were blue, and since my eyes are brown this puzzled me for many years until I was told that the eyes of all infants are blue at birth. The baby was whimpering miserably, and I could sense in him a terrible constraint and fear.

I knew that this was my own deepest fear, the fear that moved my life. I tried to find words to convince the baby not to be afraid and as I searched for the words, the experience became overwhelming. I stopped palming and lay on my bed, my eyes covered with a towel. I was firmly in the grip of my fear, but I felt a kind of relief to be in touch with it.

I began palming again, and the baby was still there. Again I asked him, "Why aren't you breathing?" This time he responded in Hebrew, "Because I am afraid to see." I had never believed in this kind of experience, and had always belittled others who spoke of them. But here I was talking with myself as a child. Though I was nearly frozen with fear myself, I tried to console him. "Don't be afraid. There is nothing to fear." Overwhelmed, I stopped palming again. I knew I was not strong enough to confront this embodiment of my deepest fear.

I left the room and took a short walk in the afternoon sun. Refreshed, I returned once again to palming, and the image of the baby was faint and slowly disappearing. I felt relaxed and open, probably from the walk. Then another image appeared. I was in Israel, in the library of Miriam, the person who led me to a life of sight. Unlike the vision of the baby which was of the past, this was clearly a vision of the future. I stood in Miriam's library, reading a book which was ten feet away. I felt a great confidence and deep satisfaction.

There is no reason I should not read from that distance. At present I am not even halfway there, but I see no more obstacles in my way.

For more information, please contact:

Center for Self-Healing
1718 Taraval Street
San Francisco CA 94116
USA

Tel: 0101-415-665-9574

ARKANA – NEW-AGE BOOKS FOR MIND, BODY AND SPIRIT

With over 150 titles currently in print, Arkana is the leading name in quality new-age books for mind, body and spirit. Arkana encompasses the spirituality of both East and West, ancient and new, in fiction and non-fiction. A vast range of interests are covered, including Psychology and Transformation, Health, Science and Mysticism, Women's Spirituality and Astrology.

If you would like a catalogue of Arkana books, please write to:

Arkana Marketing Department
Penguin Books Ltd
27 Wright's Lane
London W8 5TZ

ARKANA – NEW-AGE BOOKS FOR MIND, BODY AND SPIRIT

A selection of titles already published or in preparation

Neal's Yard Natural Remedies Susan Curtis, Romy Fraser and Irene Kohler

Natural remedies for common ailments from the pioneering Neal's Yard Apothecary Shop. An invaluable resource for everyone wishing to take responsibility for their own health, enabling you to make your own choice from homeopathy, aromatherapy and herbalism.

The Arkana Dictionary of New Perspectives Stuart Holroyd

Clear, comprehensive and compact, this iconoclastic reference guide brings together the orthodox and the highly unorthodox, doing full justice to *every* facet of contemporary thought – psychology and parapsychology, culture and counter-culture, science and so-called pseudo-science.

The Absent Father: Crisis and Creativity Alix Pirani

Freud used Oedipus to explain human nature; but Alix Pirani believes that the myth of Danae and Perseus has most to teach an age which offers 'new responsibilities for women and challenging questions for men' – a myth which can help us face the darker side of our personalities and break the patterns inherited from our parents.

Woman Awake: A Celebration of Women's Wisdom Christina Feldman

In this inspiring book, Christina Feldman suggests that it *is* possible to break out of those negative patterns instilled into us by our social conditioning as women: confirmity, passivity and surrender of self. Through a growing awareness of the dignity of all life and its connection with us, we can regain our sense of power and worth.

Water and Sexuality Michel Odent

Taking as his starting point his world-famous work on underwater childbirth at Pithiviers, Michel Odent considers the meaning and importance of water as a symbol: in the past – expressed through myths and legends – and today, from an advertisers' tool to a metaphor for aspects of the psyche. Dr Odent also boldly suggests that the human species may have had an aquatic past.